EASY EXERCISES *for* PREGNANCY

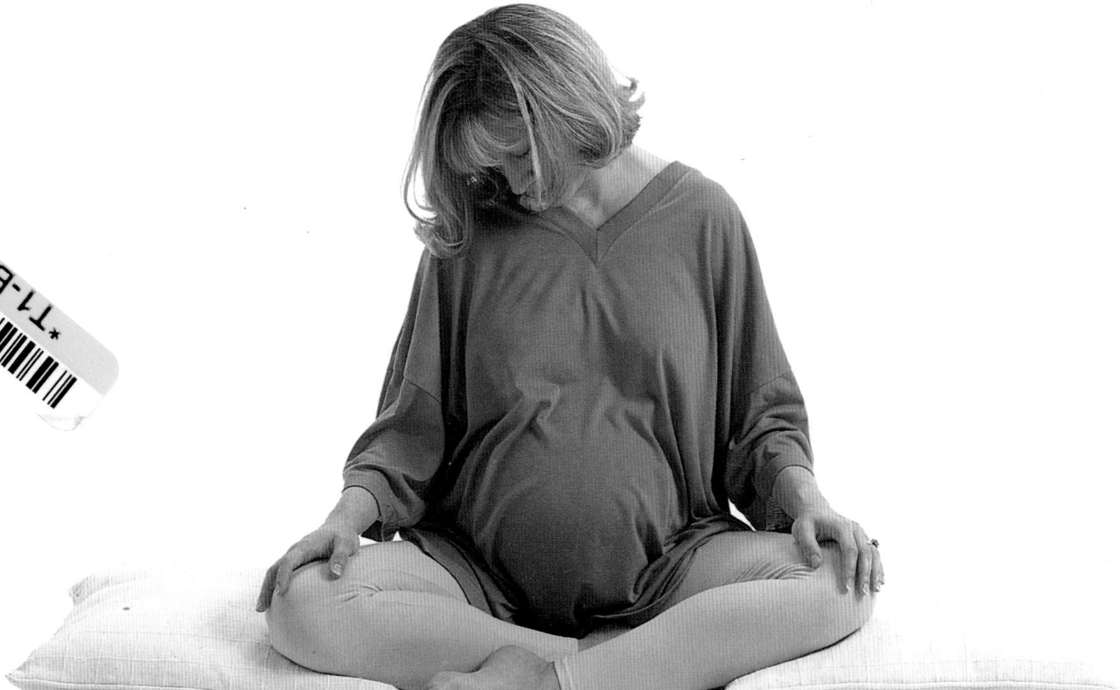

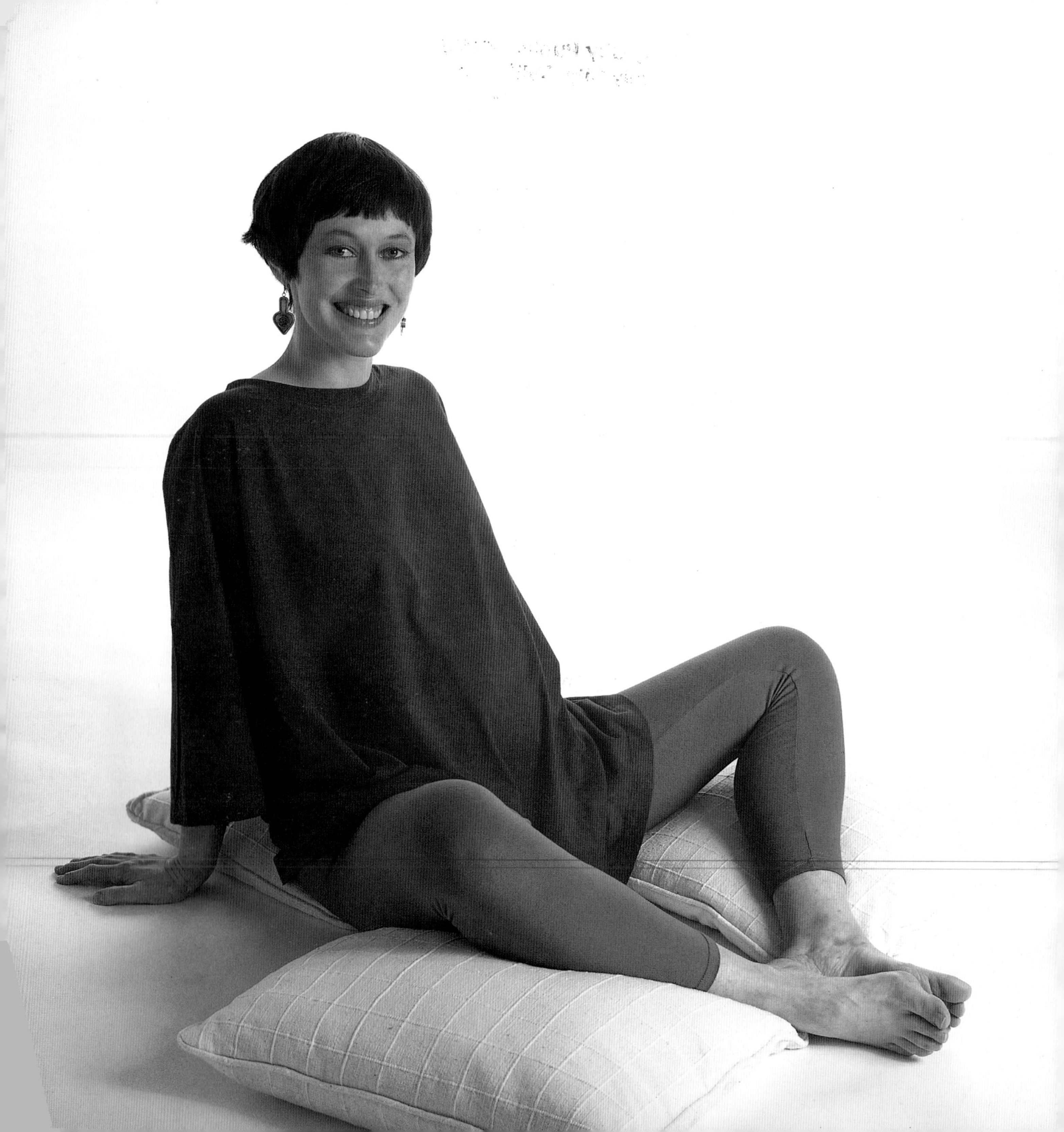

EASY EXERCISES *for* PREGNANCY

Janet Balaskas

Photographs by Anthea Sieveking

Macmillan • USA

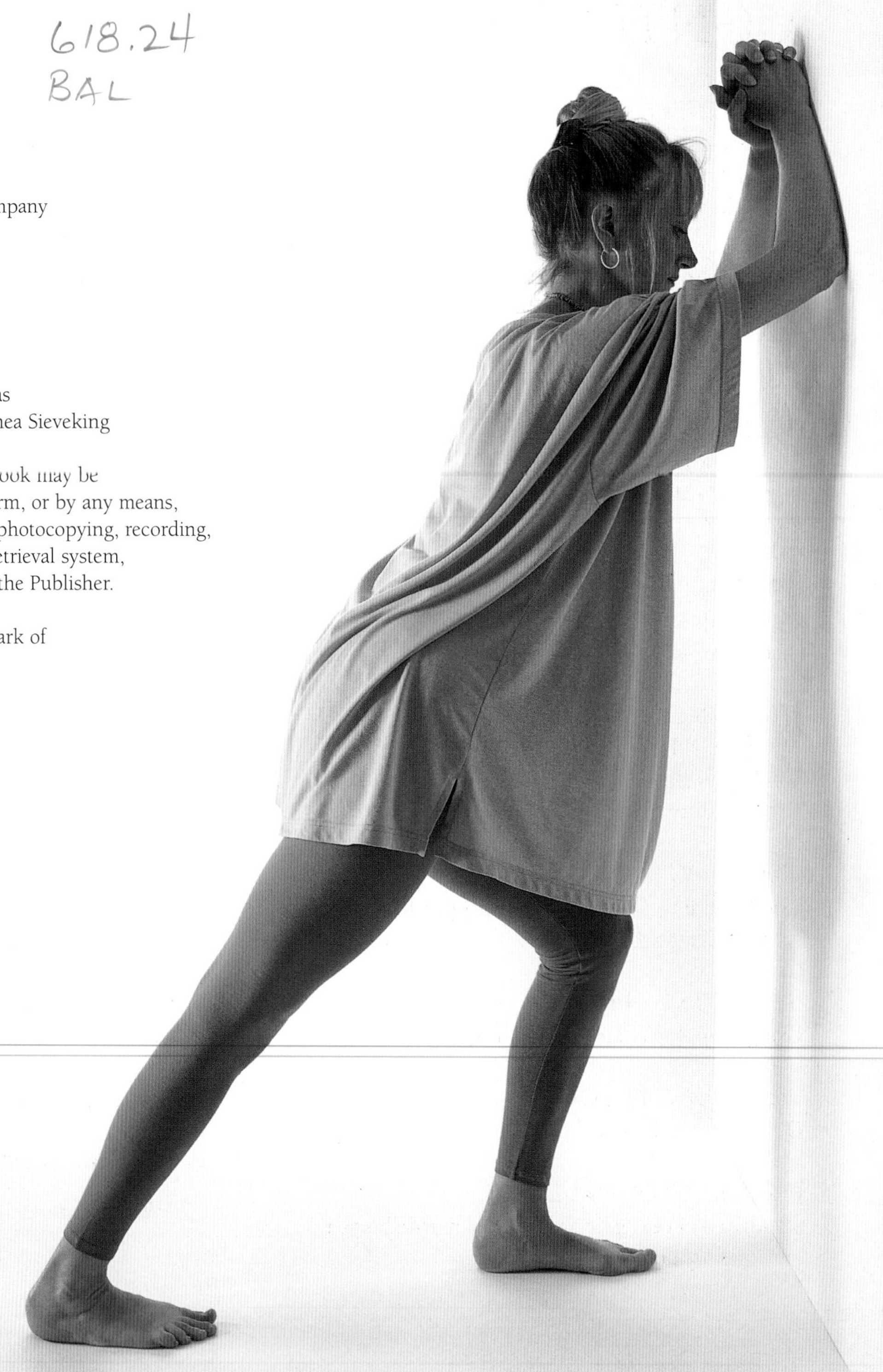

MACMILLAN
A Simon & Schuster Macmillan Company
1633 Broadway
New York, NY 10019

Easy Exercises for Pregnancy

Contact Library of Congress for full Cataloging-in-Publication Data

ISBN 0-02-861661-8

Printed in Hong Kong

10 9 8 7 6 5 4 3 2 1

CONTENTS

THE BENEFITS OF EXERCISE

Introducing a program of easy exercises into your daily life is a very positive decision. This is particularly so while you are pregnant and are faced with the challenges of carrying your growing baby and giving birth, and also as you think ahead to the postnatal months.

This book teaches you how to use your body positively, which will make a tremendous difference to your health and the way you feel while you are pregnant. It can also empower you to cope well with your labor and birth, to recover quickly afterward, and to enjoy good health and energy when caring for your baby.

You can use this exercise program regardless of whether this is your first, second, or subsequent baby, or even if you are carrying twins. Generally, the movements and positions involved are helpful for women who have back pain, sciatica, or any of the common problems that can occur in pregnancy, although it is always wise to check with your doctor or midwife and show him or her this book before you start. It is a good idea to go for a gentle walk or swim two or three times a week in addition to doing some of these exercises on a daily basis. This should be all you need to be fit and healthy throughout your pregnancy.

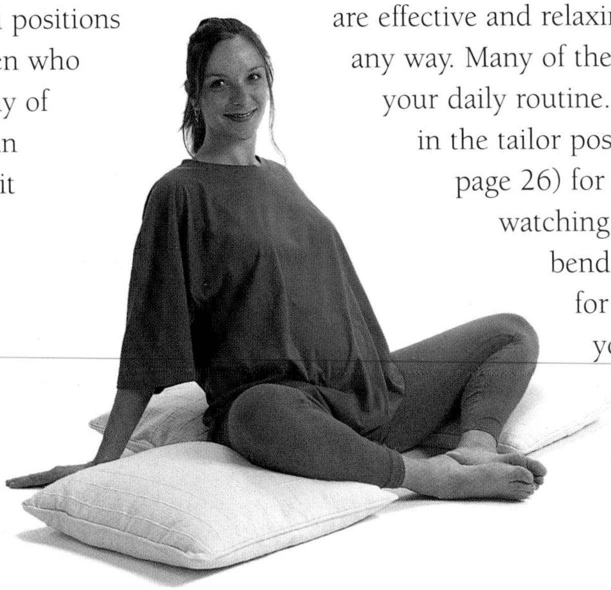

The exercises herein are especially designed for pregnancy and are based on my many years of experience teaching pregnant women. It is very important that exercise not be strenuous. This is because your heart and lungs are already working at increased levels during pregnancy, which is itself a natural kind of aerobic exercise. The last thing you need is an aerobic "workout" on top of that. However, you do need to exercise your body sensibly and to keep fit.

If you follow the instructions carefully, you will find that the exercises in this book are easy to do, as well as safe for you and your baby. They are effective and relaxing, yet not strenuous in any way. Many of the exercises can fit in with your daily routine. For example, you can sit in the tailor position shown left (and see page 26) for a few minutes while watching television, or do a forward bend (page 41) while waiting for water to boil. However, if you can find the time, it is beneficial to set aside 30 to 60 minutes a day to practice the exercises. This will give you an opportunity to unwind and relax each day and to pay attention to yourself and the vital work you are doing in nourishing your baby. This is particularly helpful if you are working during pregnancy. It will help you to cope better with even the busiest lifestyle. If you are having your second or a subsequent baby, this program may be the only time you have for yourself to recharge your energy and focus on the new baby.

Increasing energy

Many women complain about tiredness and exhaustion during pregnancy. This is not surprising since your body is working harder than usual to protect and nourish your baby. However, feeling tired is also caused by stagnant or blocked energy due to a lack of suitable exercise or poor posture. Your energy level can improve dramatically when you start to practice a few simple exercises on a regular basis. You may also find that you sleep better at night.

I always notice after an exercise class that mothers who arrive feeling exhausted are more energized and refreshed by the time they leave. The effect is cumulative, too, so that exercising regularly, in the right way, can transform the months ahead from a time of discomfort and indisposition to one in which you feel healthy, strong, and energetic.

Improving posture

Now that you are carrying a baby, your posture is more important than ever. Our modern lifestyle often results in poor postural habits that can affect us during pregnancy. For example, watching television while lying on the sofa with your feet up on the coffee table may seem relaxing, but it slows down the circulation of blood to the placenta and, especially in late pregnancy, could be forcing your baby into a less advantageous position for the birth. In fact, it is much better to sit up straight with your back well supported, or else to lie on your side or to relax leaning forward over a large cushion.

As you practice the exercises in this book, you will also be learning how to position your body when going about your daily life, whether you are standing, walking, sitting, working at a desk, resting, watching television, or sleeping. Not only will you feel much better, but also your baby will benefit from a better supply of nutrients and oxygen, and you will be doing your best to help your baby move into a good position for birth.

Encouraging flexibility and suppleness

The exercises in this book are all natural movements that our bodies are designed to execute with ease. However, because of the way we live, there are certain movements we do not make very often that can become difficult to do. Squatting or kneeling are good examples of these. Young children use these positions with ease all the time, but adults rarely engage in such movements. As a result, our joints stiffen and muscles shorten so that, when we try to squat or kneel, we may encounter resistance and pain. However, flexibility and muscle tone can be safely improved and even restored by sensible exercise.

During pregnancy, your body becomes softer and more pliable than usual, due to changes in your hormones, so you can improve flexibility much more easily. This book will guide you to do this in an easy, gentle way, using the support of cushions, a wall, a beanbag, a chair, or a stool to allow for gradual release of tension, helped along by your breathing. The exercises are enjoyable and painless, and you'll see your general physical condition improved. These benefits will last if you continue to exercise postnatally. Improving the flexibility of your pelvic joints, hips, knees, and ankles will make you feel more comfortable while using supported upright positions during labor and when you give birth.

Good breathing

The breathing exercise on page 12 teaches you to be aware of your natural breathing rhythm. You then use this rhythm in each exercise so that you learn to focus on the wave-like rise and fall of your breathing to help you relax and release tension in each position. Once you get used to doing this, you will find that your breathing flows effortlessly and your overall lung capacity improves. Your body will respond by becoming looser and more flexible, and this, combined with good posture, means better circulation for both yourself and your baby. As you help your baby to breathe better, and to get the nutrients needed for healthy growth and development, you will enhance your own vitality and health.

During labor, being able to focus on the natural rhythm of your breathing will give you a powerful tool for managing your pain as your contractions increase. You'll be able to relax and surrender to the work your uterus is doing: opening and bringing your baby into the world. Proper breathing is invaluable if you choose to go through labor without painkillers. It may also be helpful if you do opt for some intervention. Even if you have a caesarean section, knowing how to concentrate on your breathing and how to relax can make a big difference to your comfort. Being able to focus on your spontaneous breathing rhythm during contractions in labor is more effective than learning breathing techniques, especially when you are free to move and choose the most comfortable position at the same time.

Becoming "grounded"

You will notice that I often use the word "grounded" in this book. This is because the type of exercise I recommend makes you aware of the solid earth beneath you and how the force of gravity influences your posture at all times. As you get the feel of being grounded, or more in touch with the earth, you will gain a feeling of physical support and balance and, at the same time, a sense of emotional calm and equilibrium. You will find that being grounded in the lower part of your body enables you to relax and release tension in your spine, neck, and shoulders, to avoid headaches, and to cope much better with stress. You will find this to be very useful during labor, when you discover that you can release pain by breathing into the ground. There is a constant exchange during contractions in which the earth seems to absorb pain and give back fresh energy. Being grounded helps you to stay calm, relaxed, and nourished by this help from the earth, leaving your upper body free to relax and expand into the space around you.

A positive pregnancy

I believe that it is essential to do something in pregnancy that reminds you every day that there is a miracle taking place inside your body. These exercises make you feel great. They let you know that everything is going well. They help you to have confidence in your body and to approach labor optimistically and without fear.

You also have the satisfaction of knowing that you are doing your best for yourself and your baby, and making the most of this wonderful but greatly demanding time in your life.

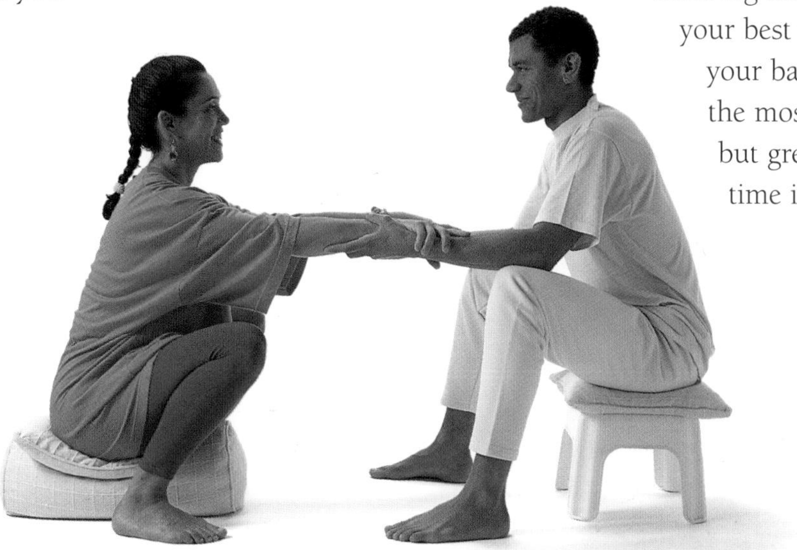

EXERCISING ON YOUR OWN

Exercising on your own is a healthy habit to develop and brings many benefits into your life. The most valuable exercise time is when you are alone so that you can concentrate on what you are doing undisturbed for 30 to 60 minutes. So the first thing you need to do is create the time.

Space and equipment

You will need a warm, uncluttered space, which includes a free stretch of wall, and some basic equipment including a simple, straight-back chair and a low stool (about ten inches high). If you can invest in a beanbag you will find it invaluable. Otherwise, three or four very large cushions will do. You will need a few small pillows as well. Some of the exercises suggest using a firm bolster, which can be obtained from a department store or futon shop. However, a rolled-up sleeping bag or two blankets rolled up into a sausage make a good substitute. You should work on a soft surface, such as a carpet or rug, or place a folded blanket underneath you.

If you sit for long periods at work, use an adjustable kneeling stool (such as the one on page 30). Or try a chair that has good back support and a seat that slopes downward. You could devise such a chair yourself by arranging two cushions on the seat so that your pelvis is slightly higher than your knees when sitting (see page 31).

Clothing

It is important to be comfortable while you exercise, so wear a big T-shirt and either comfortable leggings, loose trousers, or shorts. It is best to have bare feet for these exercises.

To begin with

Before you begin each exercise, read through all of the instructions, including the boxed sections headed "Remember." Do not worry if you cannot remember all the steps at first—you will with practice, and eventually you will only need to glance at the picture. Work through each section gradually, doing as little or as much as you want to at a time. Always begin the session with the BREATHING and BABY AWARENESS exercises (see pages 12–13), and end with a relaxation exercise (see pages 54 through 57).

You can do all of the exercises or just some of them, varying your choices throughout the week. In addition to following this program of exercises, you will benefit by going for a walk or doing some gentle swimming two or three times a week.

Aches and pains

Minor aches and pains will likely decrease once you begin to practice these exercises regularly. However, if you have back pain, sciatica, or any other serious problems, consulting a doctor who specializes in treating pregnant women is a good idea. Show your doctor this book before starting this program so that he or she can decide whether there are exercises that you should avoid. Always stop doing any exercise that causes you pain or discomfort beyond "beginner's stiffness." After a week or two, the exercises should be easy to do and completely comfortable. Though many women feel wonderful during pregnancy, others feel sick or exhausted, especially in the early months. If you are experiencing this, don't exercise too much at first, and stop if you are uneasy or any particular exercise does not feel comfortable. In time, exercising should help you to feel much better; but begin gradually, always respecting what your body is telling you. Remember, this program is not meant to be a "workout."

Listen to your body

Learning from a teacher or a book can work very well, but ultimately, your own body is your best guide to sensible exercise. Listen to what your body tells you at all times—stop if you are tired, do not do an exercise if you do not feel comfortable with it, or do more than the amount suggested if you feel up to it. Always be kind and gentle to your body, and avoid using force or pushing yourself beyond your limits. You want to end up feeling relaxed and energized, and above all you should enjoy yourself.

BREATHING

This exercise helps you to focus on your natural breathing rhythm. You can use it while doing all of the exercises in this book, as well as during labor and when breast feeding your baby.

1 Sit on the floor on the edge of a small cushion. Cross your legs comfortably and place one or two cushions under each knee so that your legs feel well supported.

2 Release your lower back downward so that your weight settles into your pelvis. Then gently lengthen your spine from the waist up to the top of your head, without arching your lower back.

3 Lengthen the back of your neck by lowering your chin slightly toward your chest. Relax your shoulders, and let your arms hang loosely by your sides, with your hands resting gently on your knees.

4 Close your eyes, and allow your eyelids and the muscles of your face to become soft and relaxed. Loosen your jaw. Focus on your breathing.

5 Breathe evenly in your natural rhythm, being aware of each time you breathe out and in.

6 Continue observing your breathing, noticing the pause between each exhalation and inhalation. Relax, take your time, and continue doing this for up to three minutes. Then, slowly open your eyes and relax.

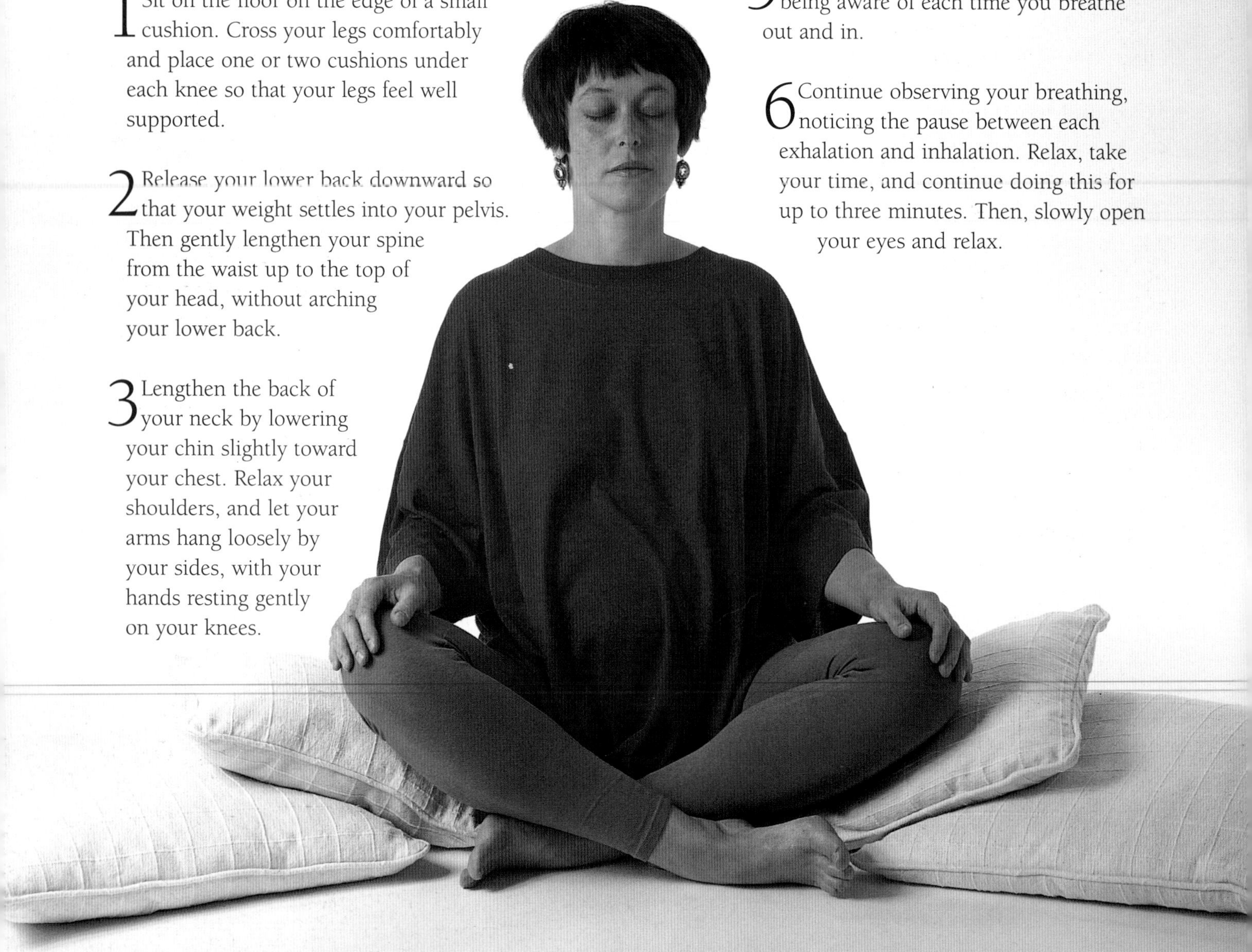

BABY AWARENESS

Sitting quietly and focusing on the rhythm of your breathing helps you to be more aware of the presence of your baby. These special times you share together are precious moments in your pregnancy.

1 Seated comfortably upright with your legs crossed, place your hands gently on your lower belly to cradle your baby. Close your eyes and relax the back of your neck, allowing your head to fall forward comfortably.

2 Focus on your breathing rhythm and then to the presence of your baby inside. Notice whether your baby is moving or lying still.

3 Now imagine what your baby is feeling and hearing—the soft sensation of warm fluid caressing the skin or the reassuring rhythm of your heart beating. Be aware of the deep connection between you and your baby, and, if you like, talk inwardly to your baby.

4 Spend the next few minutes breathing comfortably and relaxing with your baby. When you are ready, slowly return your focus to your breathing, your body, and the room around you, and then open your eyes.

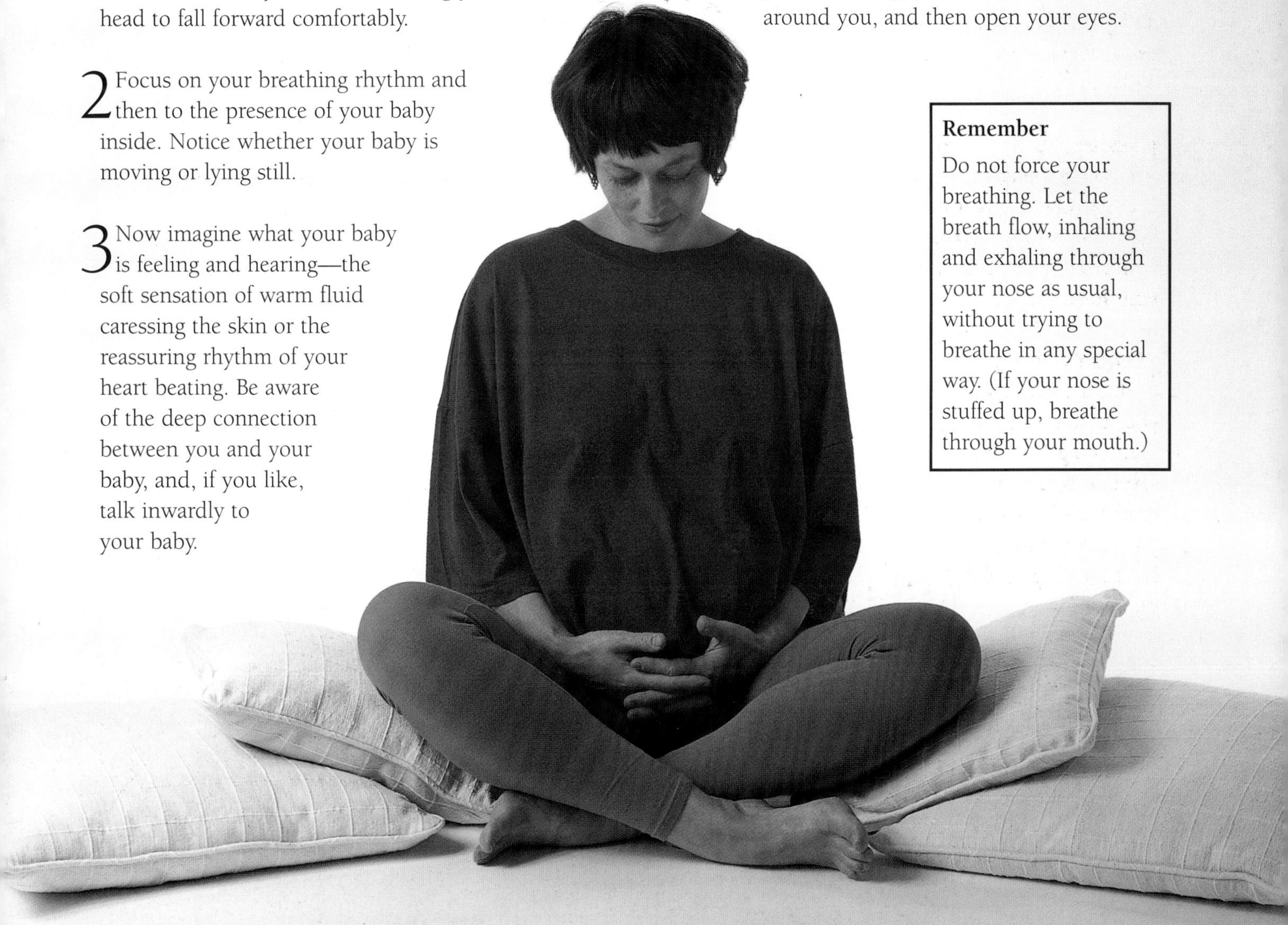

Remember

Do not force your breathing. Let the breath flow, inhaling and exhaling through your nose as usual, without trying to breathe in any special way. (If your nose is stuffed up, breathe through your mouth.)

TOES AND HEELS

The easy movements here and in the CIRCLING FEET *exercise on the opposite page improve the circulation to and from your legs, so try to do them every day.*

1 Sit on the floor with your lower back supported by a wall, or sit on the edge of a small cushion. Relax your lower back downward and then lengthen your spine. Stretch your legs out in front of you with your heels about twelve inches apart.

2 Relax your arms and shoulders and rest your hands on your thighs. Close your eyes for a moment and feel the way the backs of your legs contact the floor. Breathe evenly in your normal rhythm.

3 Open your eyes and look at your feet. Separate and wiggle your toes, and relax them.

4 Point your toes away from you. Then, as shown, extend your heels, stretching them away from you as you flex your toes toward you.

5 Alternate these two movements, first toes and then heels, and repeat ten times.

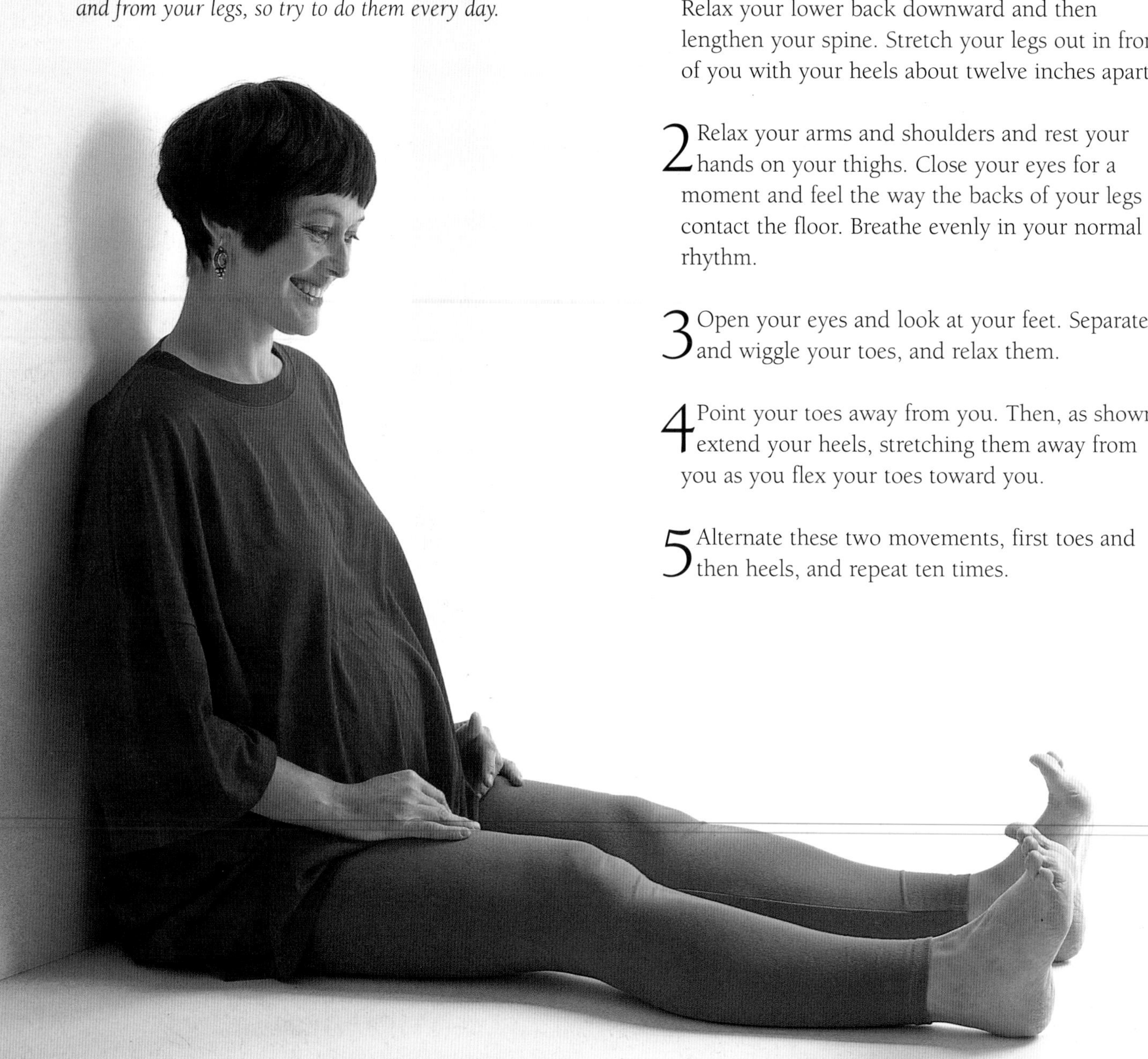

CIRCLING FEET

1 Sit against a wall or on the edge of a cushion as for the TOES AND HEELS exercise opposite.

2 Spread your legs a little wider so that your heels are about two to three feet apart. Make big, wide circles with your feet, rolling them from the ankles toward each other, and repeat ten times.

3 Now reverse the movement, circling the feet away from each other.

4 Continue circling your feet, alternating the movement from inward to outward ten times, and then relax your feet.

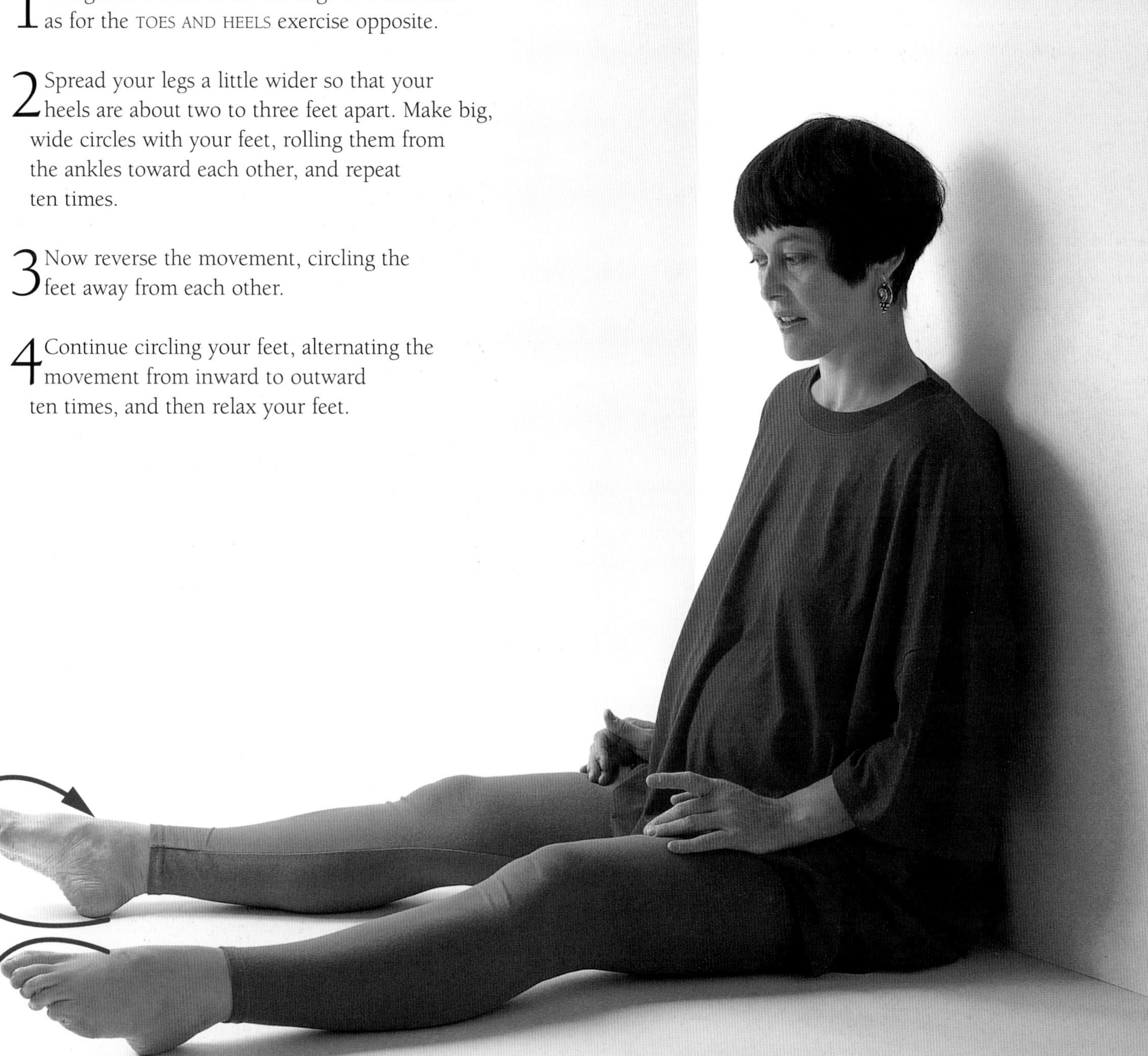

NECK ROLL

Slow, rolling movements combined with easy breathing gently release tension in the neck, jaw, and head.

1 Sit on the floor on the edge of a small cushion. Cross your legs comfortably and place a cushion or two under each knee so that your legs feel well supported.

2 Release your lower back toward the ground so that your weight settles into your pelvis. Gently lengthen your spine so that you grow tall from the waist up to your head. Do not arch your lower back.

3 Relax your shoulders, let your arms fall softly by your sides, and place your hands on your knees. Loosen your jaw and breathe evenly in your normal rhythm.

4 Keeping your back upright, slowly release your head forward to relax the muscles at the back of your neck.

5 Breathe evenly, and begin to roll your head very slowly around in big circles, releasing any tension in your neck. Continue this movement until you have completed three circles and come back to the center.

6 Pause for a second or two, notice your breathing, and repeat in the opposite direction.

7 Slowly raise your head, and return to the starting position.

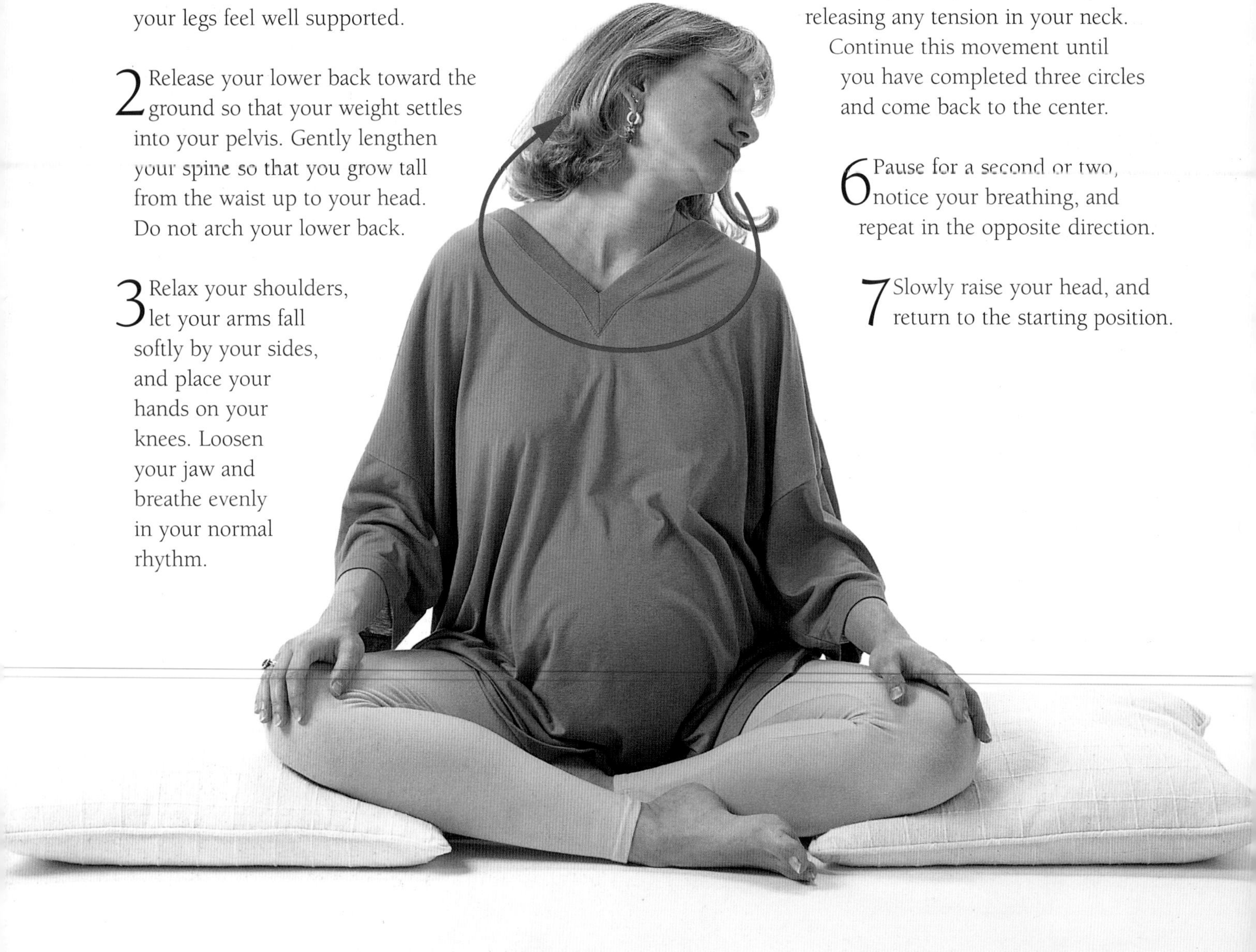

SHOULDER RELEASE

This is an exercise to loosen and relax your shoulders and to calm and "center" you.

1 Sit relaxed and do steps 1 to 3 of the NECK ROLL exercise opposite.

2 Roll your shoulders backward, making easy circular movements. Repeat this slowly, up to ten times.

3 When your shoulders feel loose, drop them back and down, creating an open feeling across the front of the chest.

4 Place the palms of your hands together, and close your eyes. Focus on your breathing, and enjoy a few minutes of inner calm. Feel how this movement makes you aware of your inner center.

5 Release your hands and open your eyes.

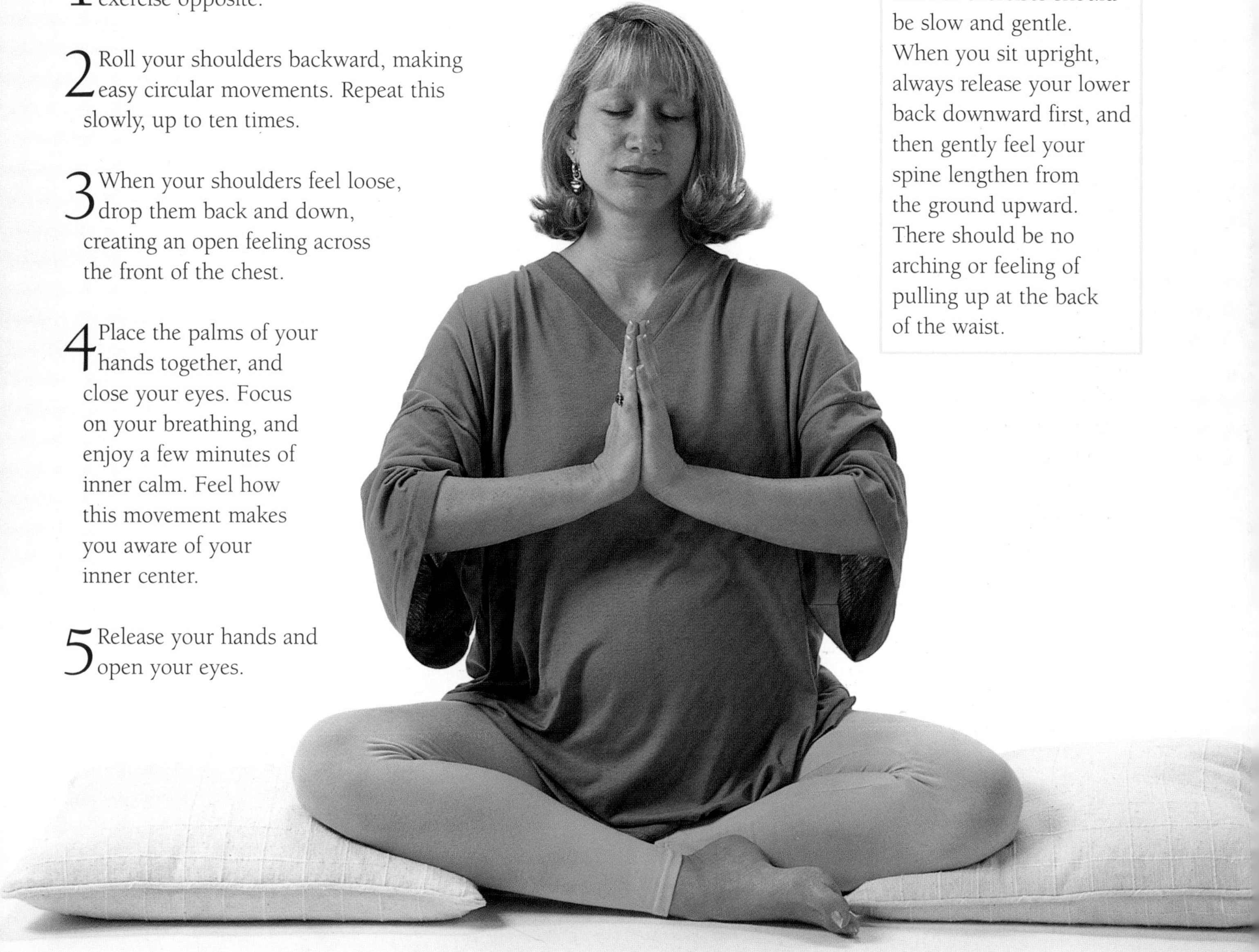

Remember

The movements in the NECK ROLL and SHOULDER RELEASE exercises should be slow and gentle. When you sit upright, always release your lower back downward first, and then gently feel your spine lengthen from the ground upward. There should be no arching or feeling of pulling up at the back of the waist.

PALM STRETCH

This is a way to release tension in the fingers, hands, and wrists, and to improve circulation to and from the hands. Repeat it three or four times.

1 Kneel on the floor on a soft surface, with a long cushion or bolster between your knees. Release the base of your spine downward. Relax your shoulders and arms, and interlock your fingers.

2 Bend your elbows, and turn your hands so that your palms are facing outward. Extend your arms, and stretch your fingers gently.

3 Breathe evenly, keeping your shoulders relaxed. Hold for about three cycles of your breathing rhythm.

4 Bend your elbows and turn your palms inward. Unclasp your hands and shake them loosely from the wrists to relax them.

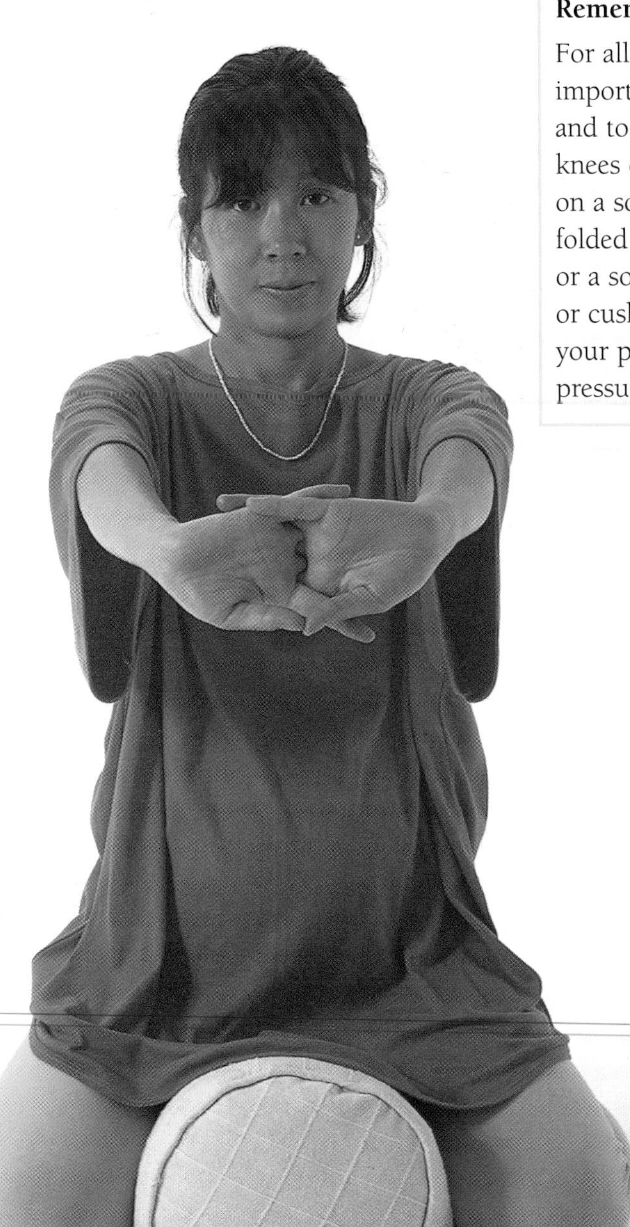

Remember

For all kneeling exercises it is important to be comfortable and to feel no strain in the knees or ankles. Always kneel on a soft surface, such as a folded blanket, an exercise mat, or a soft carpet, using a bolster or cushion if necessary to raise your pelvis. This will release pressure on the legs.

ARM RAISE

This exercise releases tension in your shoulders, with a gentle lengthening upward from the pelvis. In late pregnancy it can help to make more space for the baby, and relieve pressure under the ribs.

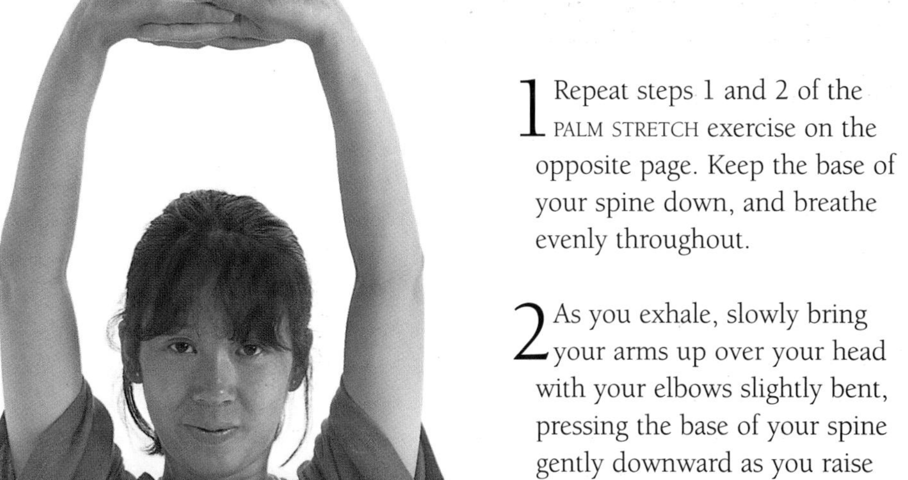

Remember

If your fingers or wrists are swollen, and they hurt when you turn your palms out, try an easier variation of both this and the previous exercise by keeping your elbows slightly bent. It is important to keep your weight centered throughout this exercise, and to avoid any arching or pulling up in the back of your waist.

1 Repeat steps 1 and 2 of the PALM STRETCH exercise on the opposite page. Keep the base of your spine down, and breathe evenly throughout.

2 As you exhale, slowly bring your arms up over your head with your elbows slightly bent, pressing the base of your spine gently downward as you raise your arms.

3 Very gently and without arching your lower back, straighten your elbows, opening your palms toward the ceiling.

4 Hold for just a few seconds, and then, as you exhale, slowly lower your arms and unclasp your hands.

5 Shake your hands gently from the wrists, and then relax.

SHOULDER RELEASE

This movement improves the flexibility of the shoulders, relieves pressure under the ribs, and improves breathing.

1 Kneel on the floor on a soft surface, with a long cushion or bolster between your legs. Sit back on your heels and relax, turning your feet inward. Release your lower back downward and settle into your pelvis.

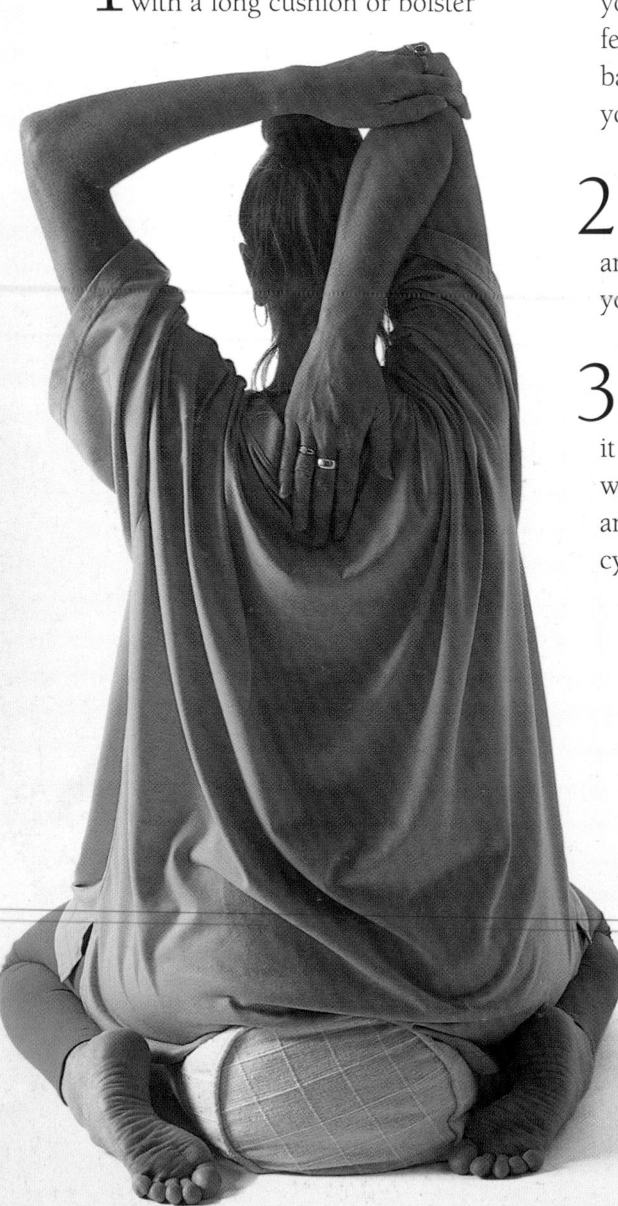

2 Slowly raise one arm up over your head. Bend your elbow, and reach down your spine with your fingers without straining.

3 Raise the other arm and catch hold of your elbow, easing it gently toward the ceiling without pulling. Breathe evenly and hold the position for three cycles of the breathing rhythm.

4 Release both arms. Rest for a moment, and repeat on the other side.

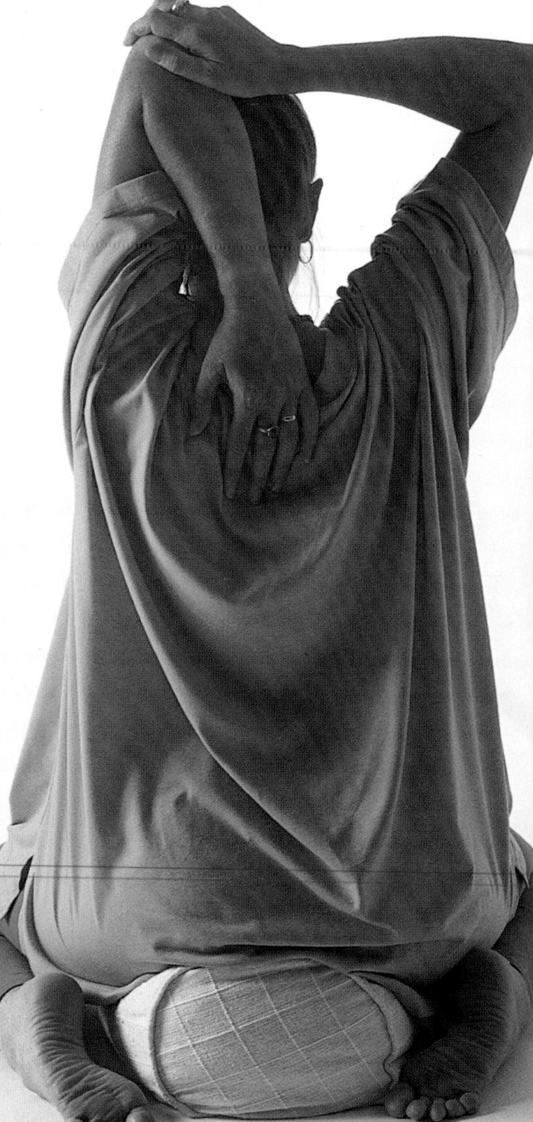

Remember

Allow the release to take place slowly as you breathe. Keep your lower back down and your neck relaxed.

SHOULDER STRETCH

This movement is ideal to practice during pregnancy and is also helpful postnatally to release tension in the shoulders after carrying or feeding your baby.

1 Kneel on the floor on a soft surface with your knees about twelve inches away from a wall. If you like, place a long cushion between your legs.

2 Spread your knees apart and turn your feet in toward each other. Sit back on your heels, drop your lower back, and settle into your pelvis.

3 Raise both arms above your head, keeping the base of your spine down. Slowly lean forward from your hips and reach up the wall, placing your palms about twelve inches apart.

4 With your arms straight, drop your weight down into your hips, gently curling your lower back toward your heels.

5 Relax the area between your shoulders until you feel a gentle stretch in your shoulders and upper arms. Breathe evenly, and hold the position for about three cycles of the breathing rhythm.

6 Release your arms and curl up slowly, first dropping your lower back down toward your feet. Gently roll your shoulders backward a few times and then repeat.

Remember

Keep your lower back and pelvis down. Press your tailbone toward your feet to avoid arching your back, and breathe comfortably in your normal rhythm.

SPREADING OUT

This movement makes you feel wide as well as long in your upper body, providing plenty of space for your baby. You can practice the exercise either sitting on the floor as shown, or seated upright in a chair to increase your awareness of your posture throughout the day.

1 Sit in the starting position given on page 16. (You might like to refold your legs with the other one in front.) Release your lower back downward, and then lengthen your spine gently from the back of the waist up to the top of your head.

2 Extend your arms sideways and touch the ground very lightly with your fingertips. As you lift your hands slowly off the ground, make tiny "flying" movements in slow motion.

3 Open your arms gently outward on either side of your body, like a pair of wings unfolding. Slowly lift your arms until they reach the height of your shoulders.

4 Keep your shoulders and wrists relaxed. Hold for a few seconds and breathe evenly in your normal rhythm.

5 Slowly release your arms down toward the ground, until your hands are resting softly on the cushions.

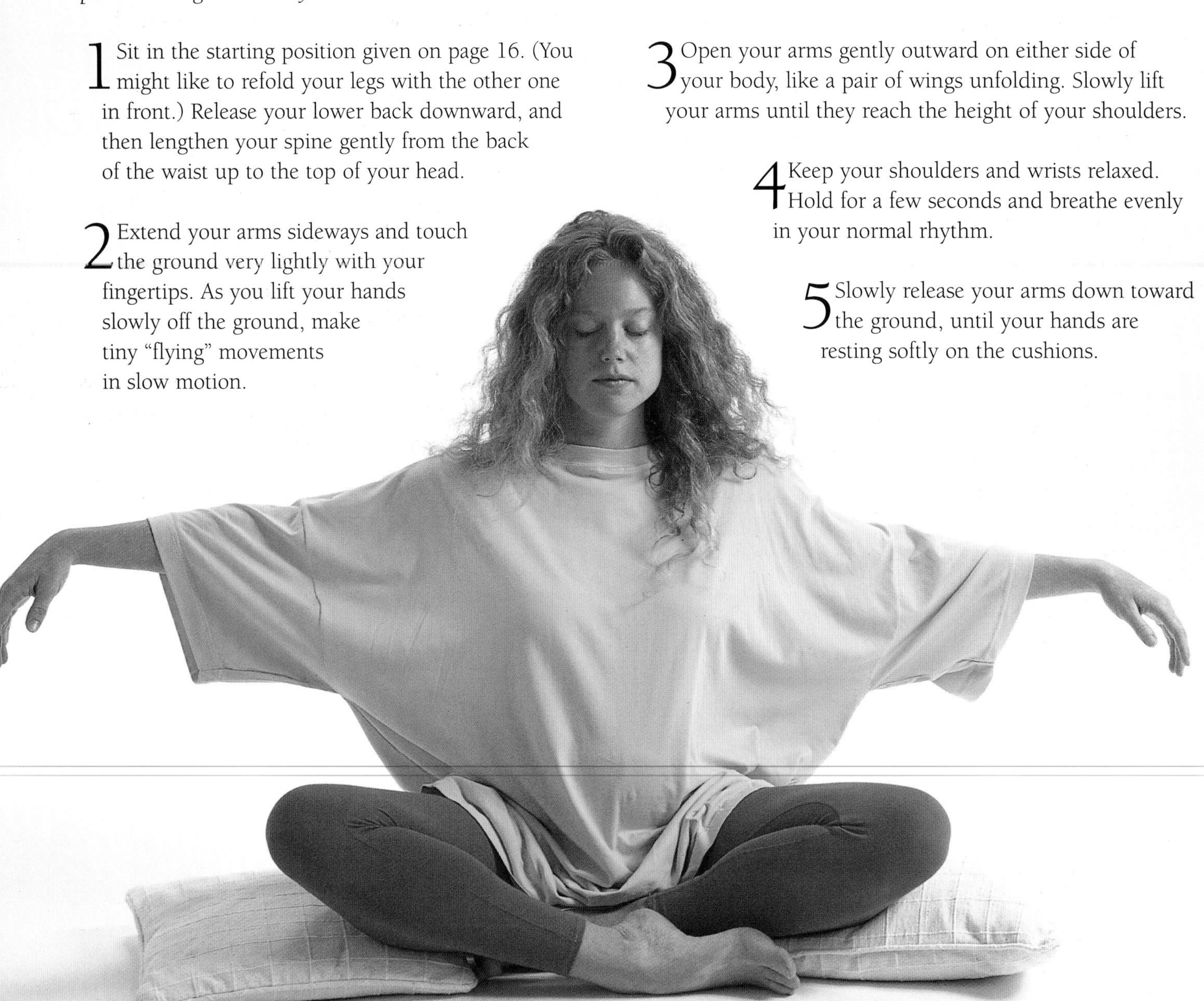

GENTLE SITTING TWIST

This gentle turning helps to maintain flexibility of the spine and releases muscular tension in the upper back, neck, and shoulders.

1 Remain seated in the same position as in the SPREADING OUT exercise on the opposite page and place your hands gently on your knees.

2 Release the base of your spine down toward the floor. Feel your spine lengthen from the waist up your neck and to the top of your head. Be aware of the rhythm of your breathing.

Remember

The turning movement should be slow and gentle, allowing time for your body to relax into the position as you breathe. Keep your spine vertical with your lower back pressing downward throughout.

3 As if the movement is coming from the ground, very slowly turn your upper body toward the left, keeping your spine vertical.

4 Bring your right arm across your body and hold your right thigh on or just above the knee. Relax your left arm from the shoulder, and touch the floor lightly behind you without leaning back; if your hand does not reach the floor, place it behind your back.

5 Continue turning your upper body to the left until your head looks over your left shoulder.

6 Hold for three cycles of your normal breathing rhythm. Then, move back slowly to the center and repeat on the other side.

LEG SPREAD

This exercise helps you to feel "grounded" through the pelvis and legs, like a tree with roots, while your spine and upper body feel light and free.

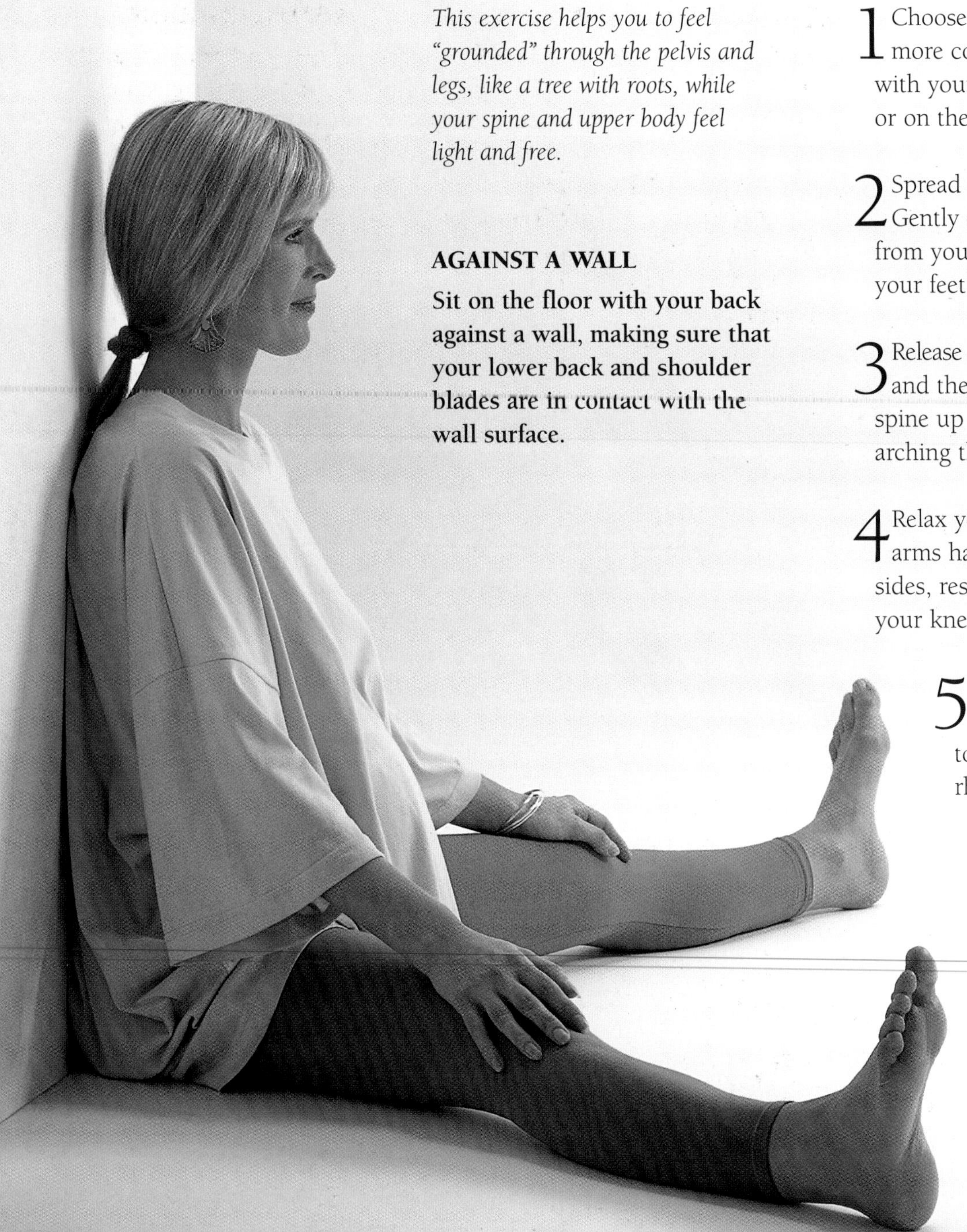

AGAINST A WALL

Sit on the floor with your back against a wall, making sure that your lower back and shoulder blades are in contact with the wall surface.

1 Choose whichever position feels more comfortable, sitting either with your back supported by a wall or on the edge of a small cushion.

2 Spread your legs comfortably apart. Gently extend your heels away from your body and then relax your feet.

3 Release your lower back downward, and then gently lengthen your spine up toward your neck without arching the back of your waist.

4 Relax your shoulders, and let your arms hang down loosely by your sides, resting your hands gently on your knees.

5 Then, with your eyes open or closed, take a moment to focus on your breathing rhythm.

Remember

Use this position every day. Avoid straining by opening your legs too wide—comfortably wide is good enough!

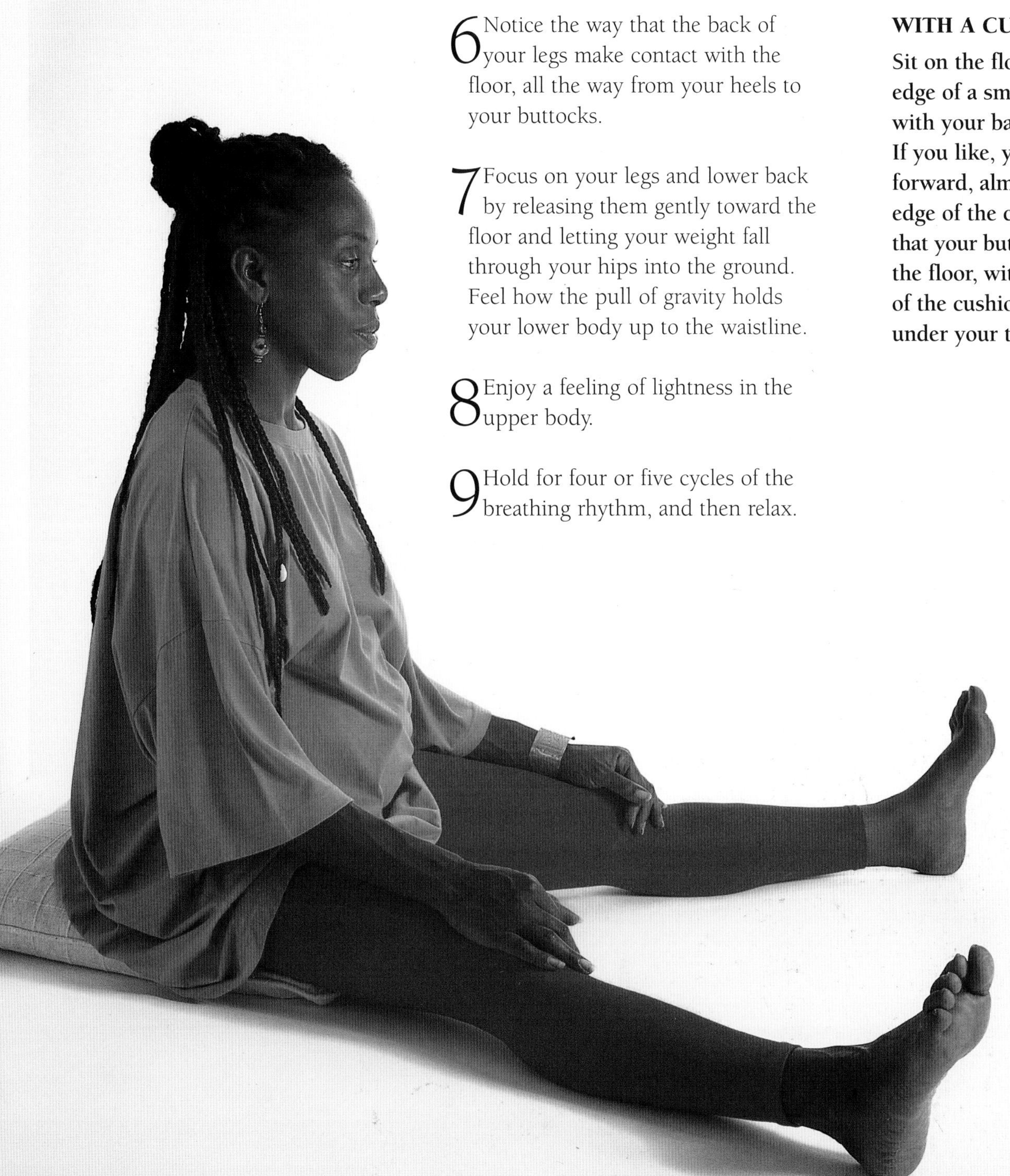

6 Notice the way that the back of your legs make contact with the floor, all the way from your heels to your buttocks.

7 Focus on your legs and lower back by releasing them gently toward the floor and letting your weight fall through your hips into the ground. Feel how the pull of gravity holds your lower body up to the waistline.

8 Enjoy a feeling of lightness in the upper body.

9 Hold for four or five cycles of the breathing rhythm, and then relax.

WITH A CUSHION

Sit on the floor on the edge of a small cushion with your back upright. If you like, you can slide forward, almost off the edge of the cushion, so that your buttocks are on the floor, with the edge of the cushion tucked under your tailbone.

TAILOR POSITION

Tailor sitting is one of the most beneficial exercises for pregnancy. It encourages a feeling of openness in the pelvis, helps to release tension in the groin, and improves flexibility of the hip joints. In addition, circulation to the pelvic area will improve, and the pelvic floor muscles will relax and release. The natural widening of the pelvis is gently encouraged, making it easier for your baby's head to engage in late pregnancy. If you suffer from back pain, always practice tailor sitting with your lower back supported by a wall.

1 Bend both knees and bring your feet together, placing them at a comfortable distance from your body.

2 Place the soles of your feet together so that the outside edges of your feet are touching.

3 Softly release your lower back downward, and then, while keeping it down, gently lengthen your spine from your waist to the top of your head.

USING CUSHIONS

Place a cushion or two underneath each knee so that your legs are well supported.

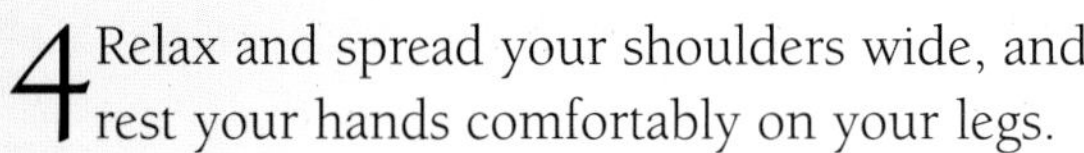

4 Relax and spread your shoulders wide, and rest your hands comfortably on your legs.

5 Relax the back of your neck and your jaw, breathe evenly, and hold the position for up to five minutes.

6 Bring your knees together gently, using your hands, to come out of the position.

Remember

Keep your feet a short distance away from your body so that you do not strain your groin. Avoid pushing or bouncing the knees. If you have pain in your pubic area, use extra cushions and place your feet further from your body, or avoid this exercise altogether.

WITHOUT CUSHIONS

You may prefer to do this exercise without cushions. But if you ever do not feel completely comfortable like this, cushions will provide your knees with extra support.

LEG SPREAD—LEANING BACK

Leaning back in this exercise and the one on the opposite page allows you to let go of your legs and to relax your lower back. This encourages the release of tension in your legs and groin and the feeling of being grounded, once you return to the upright position.

1 Sit in the LEG SPREAD position (page 24) with or without a cushion, but away from the wall. Lean back slightly and support your upper body with your arms, placing your hands on the floor behind you.

2 Relax your shoulders and the back of your neck. Gently widen and open your chest so that your breathing can flow evenly. Press your lower back downward toward the floor.

3 Close your eyes for a moment or two and relax your legs completely, letting them sink to the ground.

4 Focus on your breathing rhythm and on the contact your body makes with the ground.

5 Remain in the position for four or five cycles of the breathing rhythm, and then open your eyes and slowly sit upright.

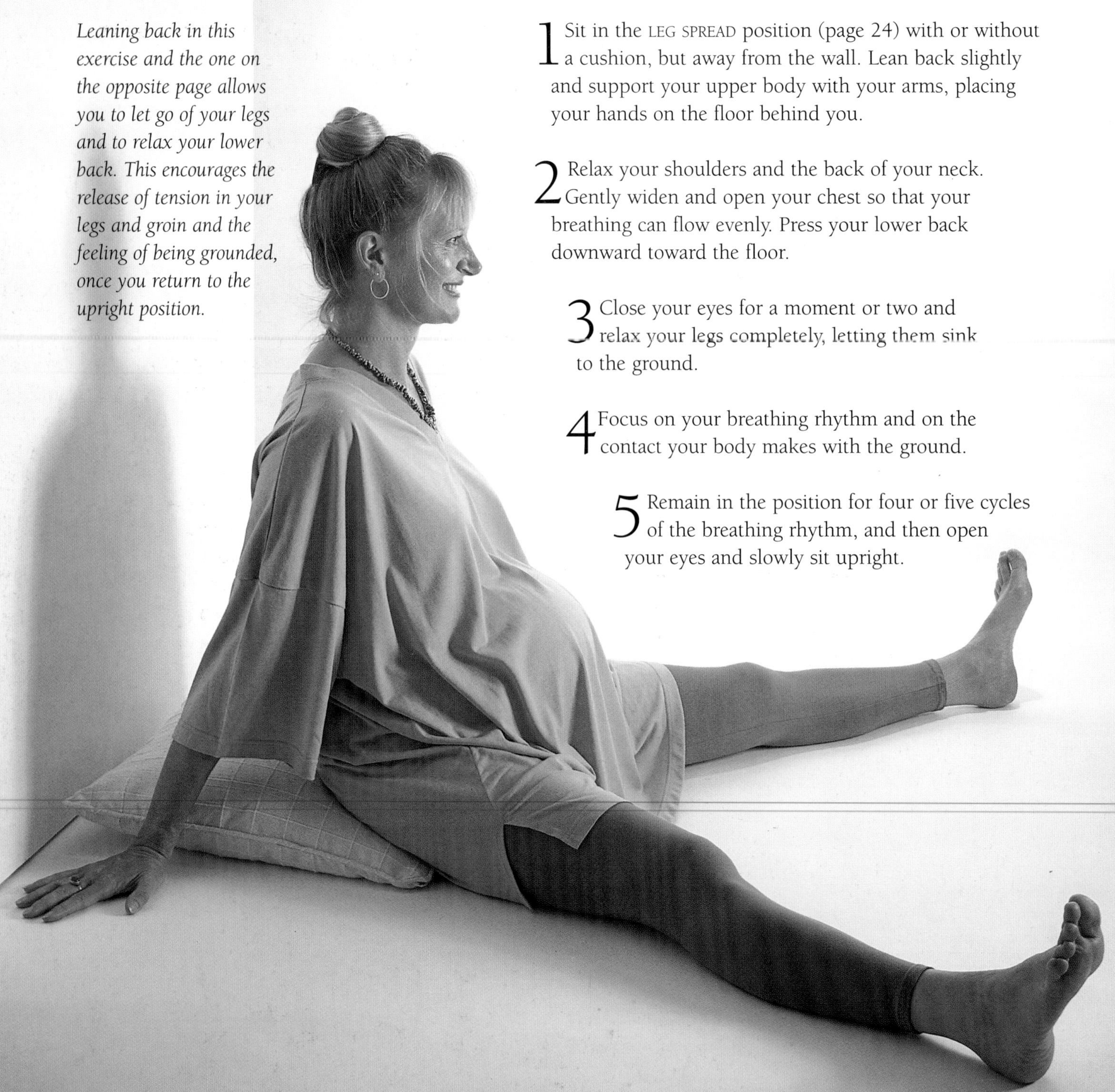

TAILOR POSITION—LEANING BACK

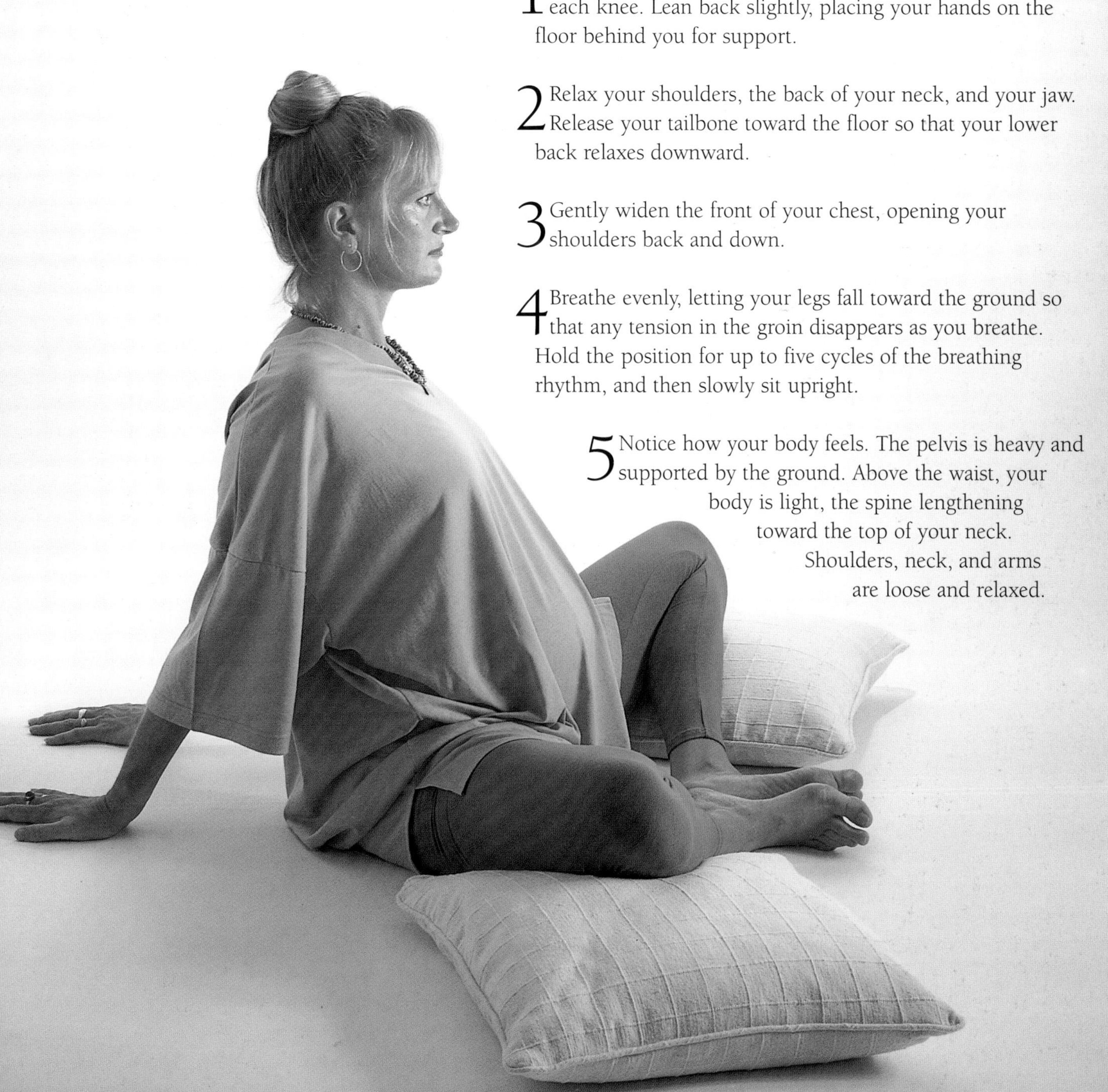

1 Sit in the TAILOR POSITION (page 26), with a cushion under each knee. Lean back slightly, placing your hands on the floor behind you for support.

2 Relax your shoulders, the back of your neck, and your jaw. Release your tailbone toward the floor so that your lower back relaxes downward.

3 Gently widen the front of your chest, opening your shoulders back and down.

4 Breathe evenly, letting your legs fall toward the ground so that any tension in the groin disappears as you breathe. Hold the position for up to five cycles of the breathing rhythm, and then slowly sit upright.

5 Notice how your body feels. The pelvis is heavy and supported by the ground. Above the waist, your body is light, the spine lengthening toward the top of your neck. Shoulders, neck, and arms are loose and relaxed.

GOOD SITTING

This exercise can be done while you are working at a desk or sitting at the dinner table. By paying attention throughout the day to your posture while sitting, you can prevent strain in your lower back and keep your neck and shoulders relaxed. In late pregnancy, a proper sitting posture can help your baby to lie in a good position.

1 Sit on a chair or kneeling stool, making sure that it is comfortable and at the right height for the desk or table. You should be able to use your arms freely while keeping your shoulders relaxed and spine upright.

2 Feel the way your body weight falls through your buttocks onto the seat, and softly release your lower back downward so that you feel securely "grounded" in the pelvis.

3 Gently lengthen your spine from the back of your waist to the top of your head, without arching or pulling up in your lower back. Relax your stomach muscles.

4 Relax your shoulders by opening them wide across the front of your chest and releasing them back and down.

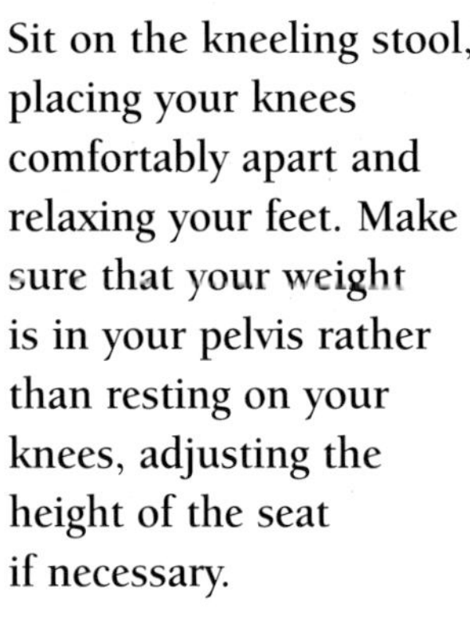

USING A KNEELING STOOL

Sit on the kneeling stool, placing your knees comfortably apart and relaxing your feet. Make sure that your weight is in your pelvis rather than resting on your knees, adjusting the height of the seat if necessary.

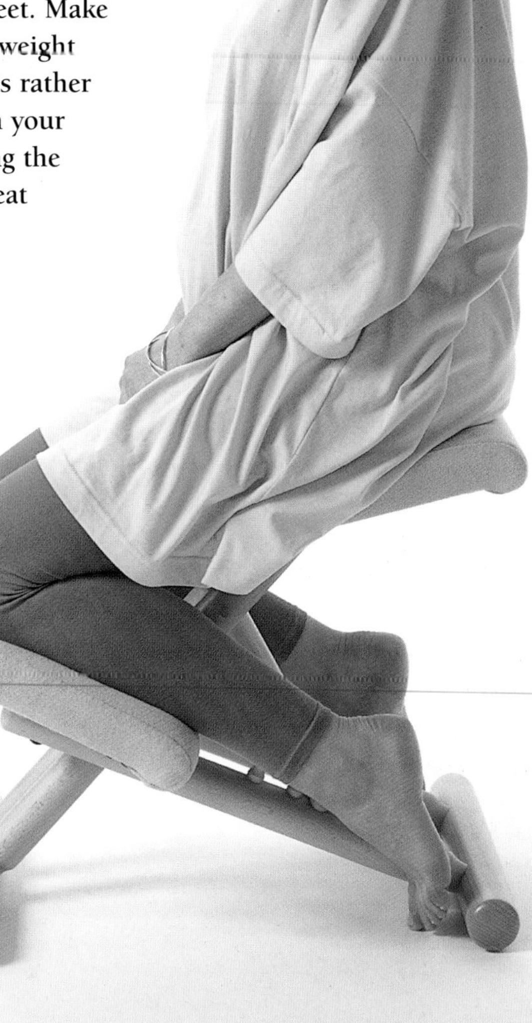

5 Raise your breast bone slightly to make space for your baby, and relax your arms.

6 Relax the back of your neck and your jaw, allowing your head to find its balance. Breathe evenly in your normal rhythm.

Remember

Avoid spending more than half an hour sitting at a time.

Get up and walk around for a few minutes if your work involves long hours at a desk. Every now and again, close your eyes for a few moments to focus on the rhythm of your breathing and the presence of your baby.

SITTING ON A CHAIR

Choose a chair which allows you to sit with your feet flat on the floor so that your legs are relaxed. Place one or two cushions on the seat of the chair to raise your pelvis so that it's a little higher than your knees. Sit far back on the chair so that the base of your spine is supported by the back of the chair, or use a cushion to avoid leaning back.

Separate your knees, and position your feet so that they can comfortably rest flat on the floor with your heels down.

Avoid crossing your legs when sitting on a chair.

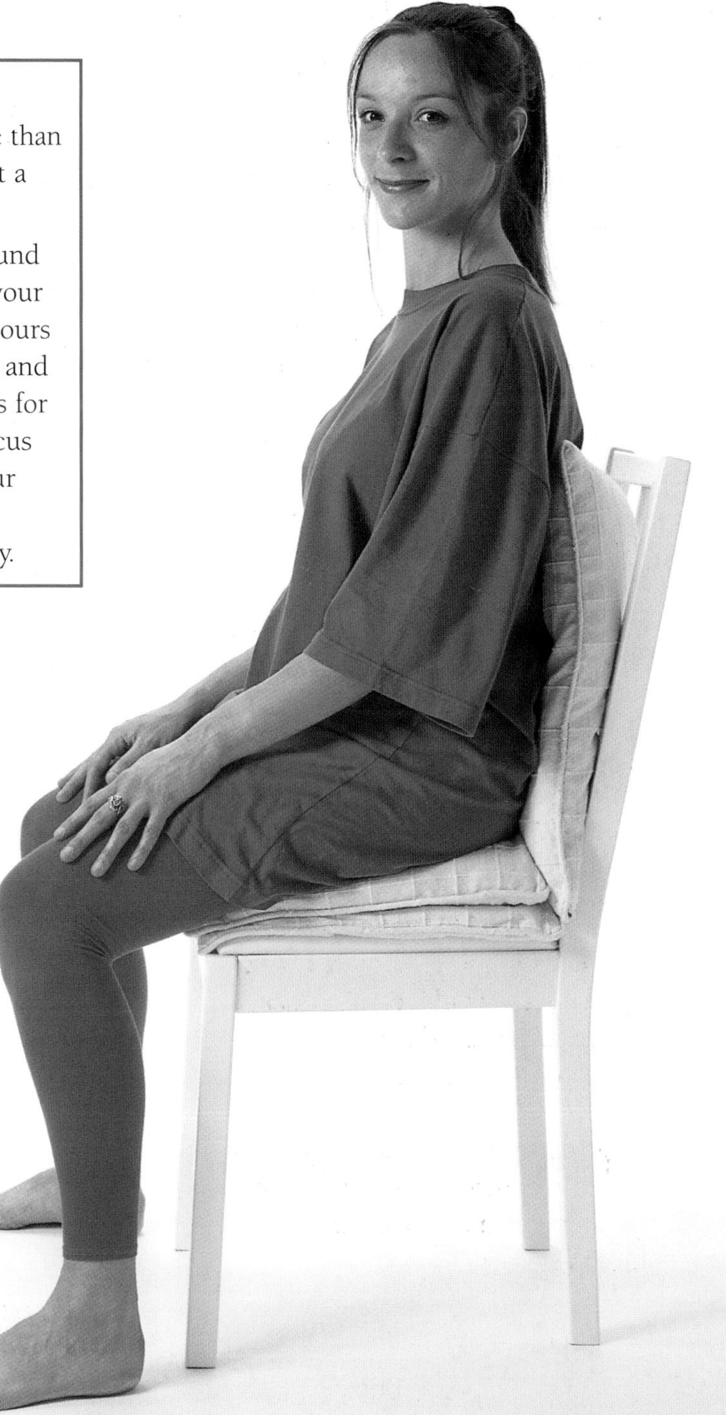

UPRIGHT CHILD'S POSE

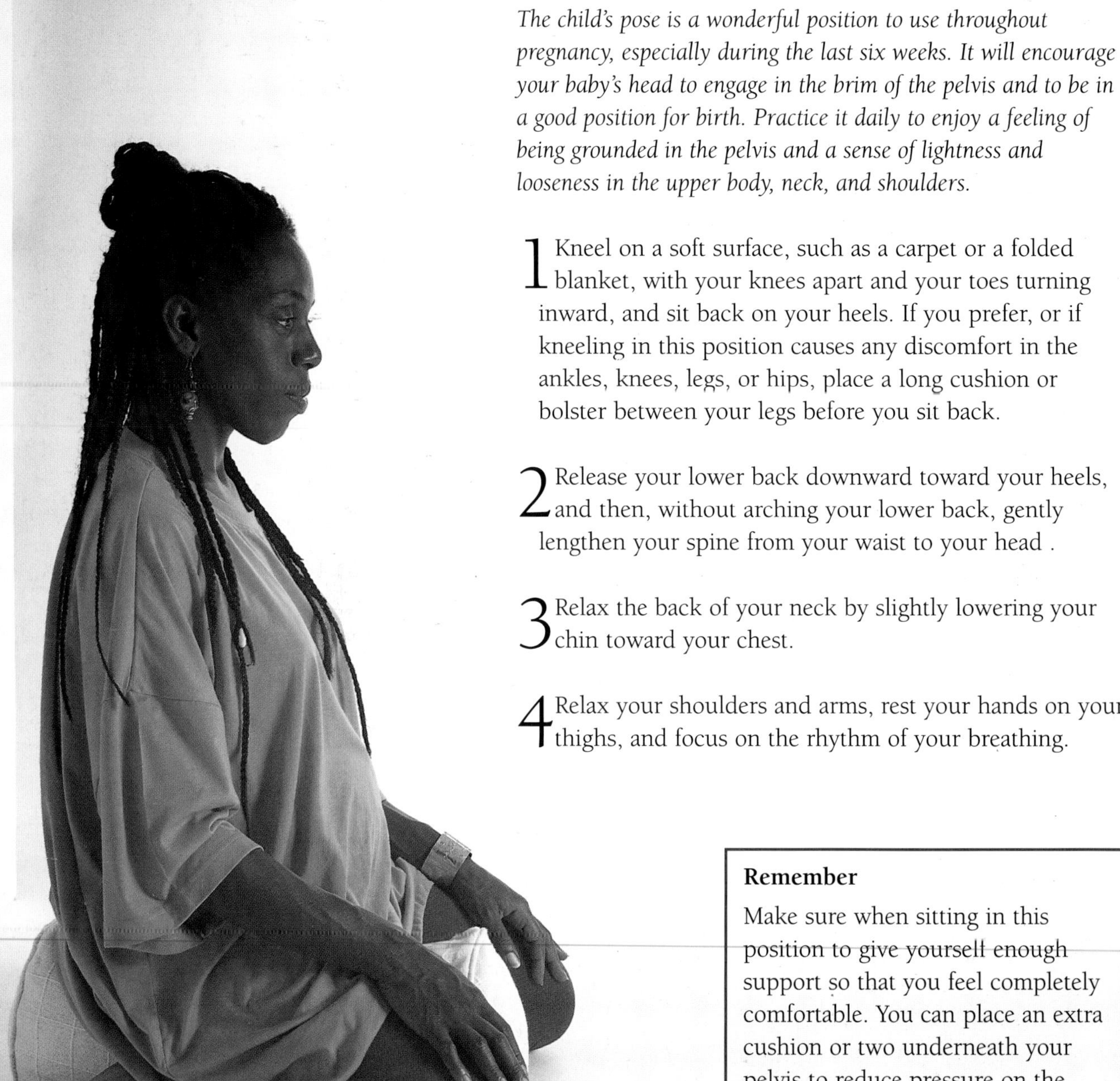

The child's pose is a wonderful position to use throughout pregnancy, especially during the last six weeks. It will encourage your baby's head to engage in the brim of the pelvis and to be in a good position for birth. Practice it daily to enjoy a feeling of being grounded in the pelvis and a sense of lightness and looseness in the upper body, neck, and shoulders.

1 Kneel on a soft surface, such as a carpet or a folded blanket, with your knees apart and your toes turning inward, and sit back on your heels. If you prefer, or if kneeling in this position causes any discomfort in the ankles, knees, legs, or hips, place a long cushion or bolster between your legs before you sit back.

2 Release your lower back downward toward your heels, and then, without arching your lower back, gently lengthen your spine from your waist to your head .

3 Relax the back of your neck by slightly lowering your chin toward your chest.

4 Relax your shoulders and arms, rest your hands on your thighs, and focus on the rhythm of your breathing.

Remember

Make sure when sitting in this position to give yourself enough support so that you feel completely comfortable. You can place an extra cushion or two underneath your pelvis to reduce pressure on the knees, calves, or ankles—this is especially important if you have painful swelling.

LENGTHENING

This exercise allows you to be aware of your spine lengthening in two directions at the same time—from the waist down toward the ground, and up toward the sky.

1 Start in the UPRIGHT CHILD'S POSE on the opposite page, with or without the long cushion or bolster. Focus on the grounded base of your spine, paying attention to your breathing.

2 Gently release your lower back downward and slowly begin to raise your arms.

3 Allow your arms to come up over your head and release your lower back downward.

4 Relax your shoulders downward as your arms lengthen toward the ceiling. Keep your wrists loose, and hold the position for two to three cycles of the normal breathing rhythm.

5 With your arms still raised, progress directly to the LEANING FORWARD exercise on the next page, or instead lower your arms gently and relax.

Remember

Keep your weight centered in your pelvis and avoid arching the back of your waist. Keep your arms and shoulders loose and relaxed as you lengthen your torso from the grounded base of your spine upward—think of growing upward like a plant from its roots toward the light.

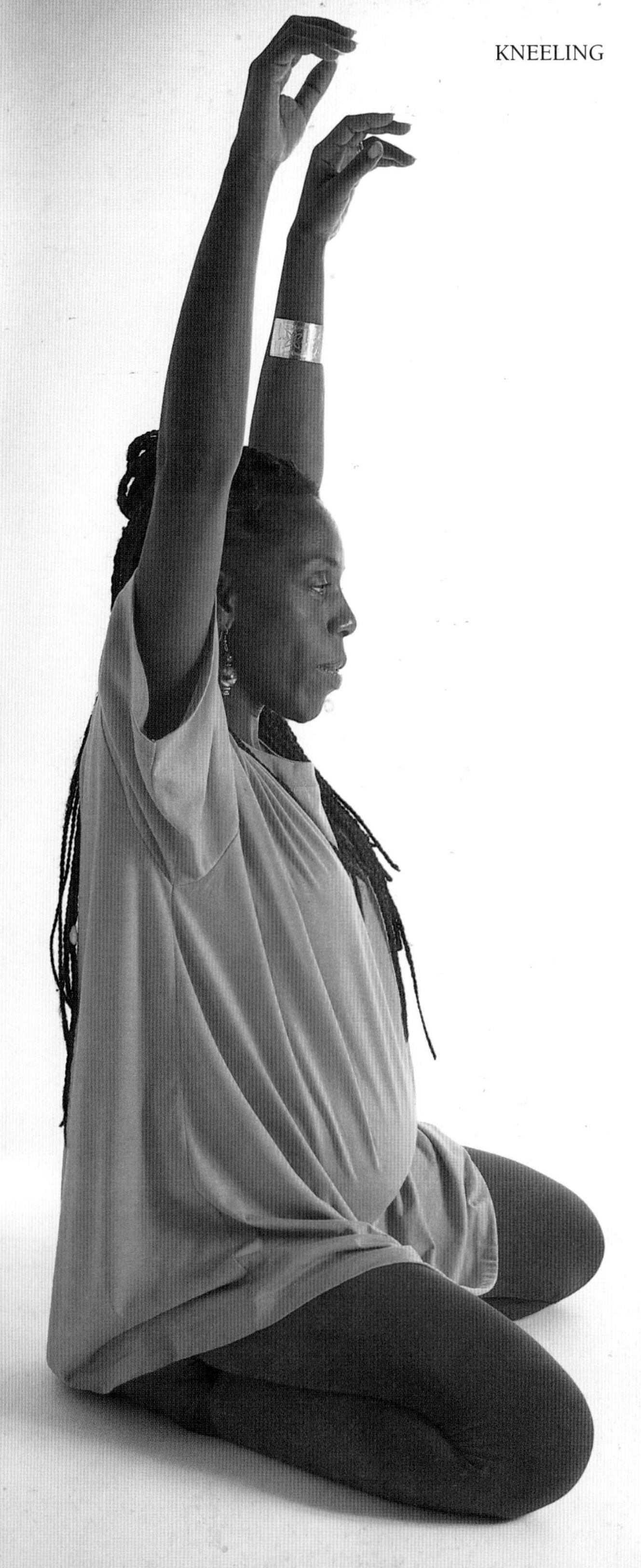

LEANING FORWARD

This movement gently tips your pelvis forward from the hips, taking the weight of your baby off your lower back. It encourages your baby to find a good position in the womb, and improves flexibility in your hips, knees, and ankles.

Remember

Your spine should feel loose and relaxed and it should not be bending—the forward movement comes from your hips. Your pelvis should rest on your heels, or on the bolster if you are using one.

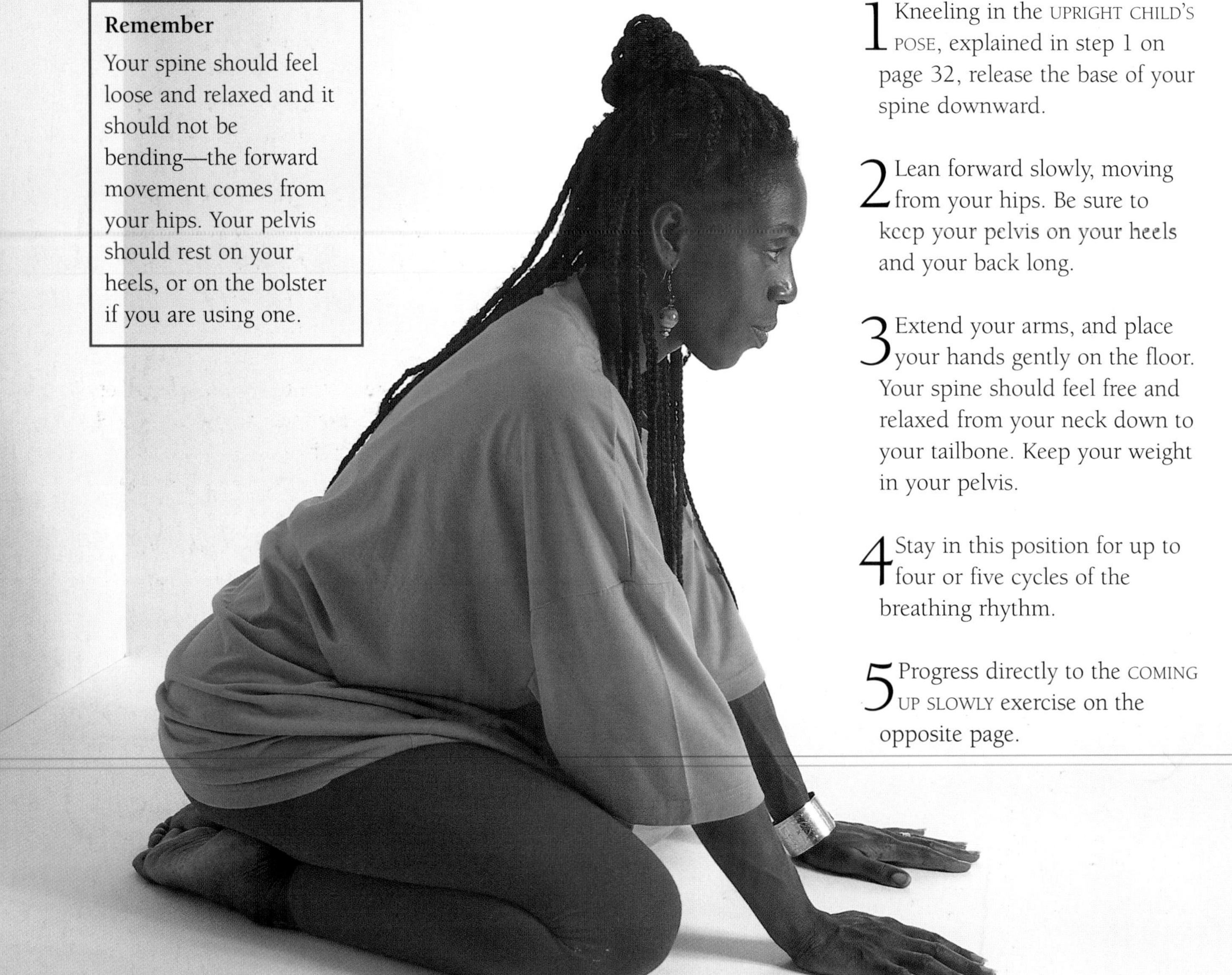

1 Kneeling in the UPRIGHT CHILD'S POSE, explained in step 1 on page 32, release the base of your spine downward.

2 Lean forward slowly, moving from your hips. Be sure to keep your pelvis on your heels and your back long.

3 Extend your arms, and place your hands gently on the floor. Your spine should feel free and relaxed from your neck down to your tailbone. Keep your weight in your pelvis.

4 Stay in this position for up to four or five cycles of the breathing rhythm.

5 Progress directly to the COMING UP SLOWLY exercise on the opposite page.

COMING UP SLOWLY

Use this exercise to return to UPRIGHT CHILD'S POSE *(page 32) whenever you come up from kneeling forward. This will help you to keep your center of gravity in the pelvis and protect your spine. Once you are upright, you will enjoy a feeling of lightness in the upper body, neck, and shoulders.*

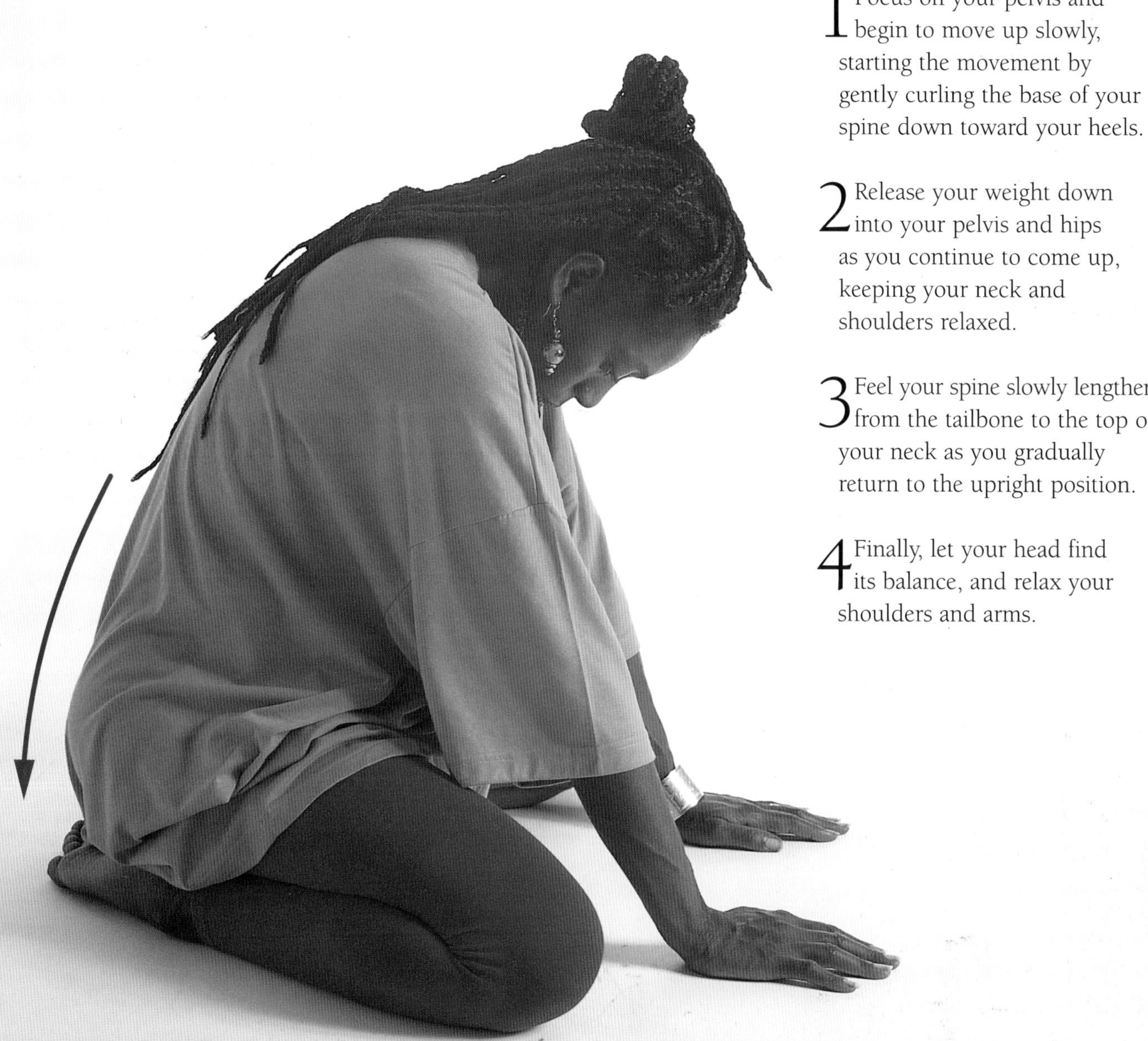

1 Focus on your pelvis and begin to move up slowly, starting the movement by gently curling the base of your spine down toward your heels.

2 Release your weight down into your pelvis and hips as you continue to come up, keeping your neck and shoulders relaxed.

3 Feel your spine slowly lengthen from the tailbone to the top of your neck as you gradually return to the upright position.

4 Finally, let your head find its balance, and relax your shoulders and arms.

RESTING OVER A BEANBAG

When you are in this position, the weight of your baby falls forward, allowing your spine to relax completely, which can help to ease or prevent backache. In late pregnancy, spending a little time every day in this position can help your baby to find the best position for birth.

1 Place a large beanbag or a few large cushions in front of you on the floor. Kneel in UPRIGHT CHILD'S POSE (page 32), using a bolster if kneeling dirctly on the floor is uncomfortable, with the beanbag close to your knees.

2 Gently press the base of your spine downward. Slowly lean forward from your hips, keeping your pelvis on your heels. Relax onto the beanbag so that your upper body is completely supported and your spine feels free.

3 Make yourself comfortable, spreading your shoulders and placing your arms loosely on the beanbag. Rest your head so that your neck is in line with the rest of your spine.

4 Close your eyes, and focus your awareness on the rhythm of your breathing and on the heaviness of your spine. Spend about five minutes relaxing in this position.

5 Return to the upright position using steps 1 to 4 in COMING UP SLOWLY, page 35.

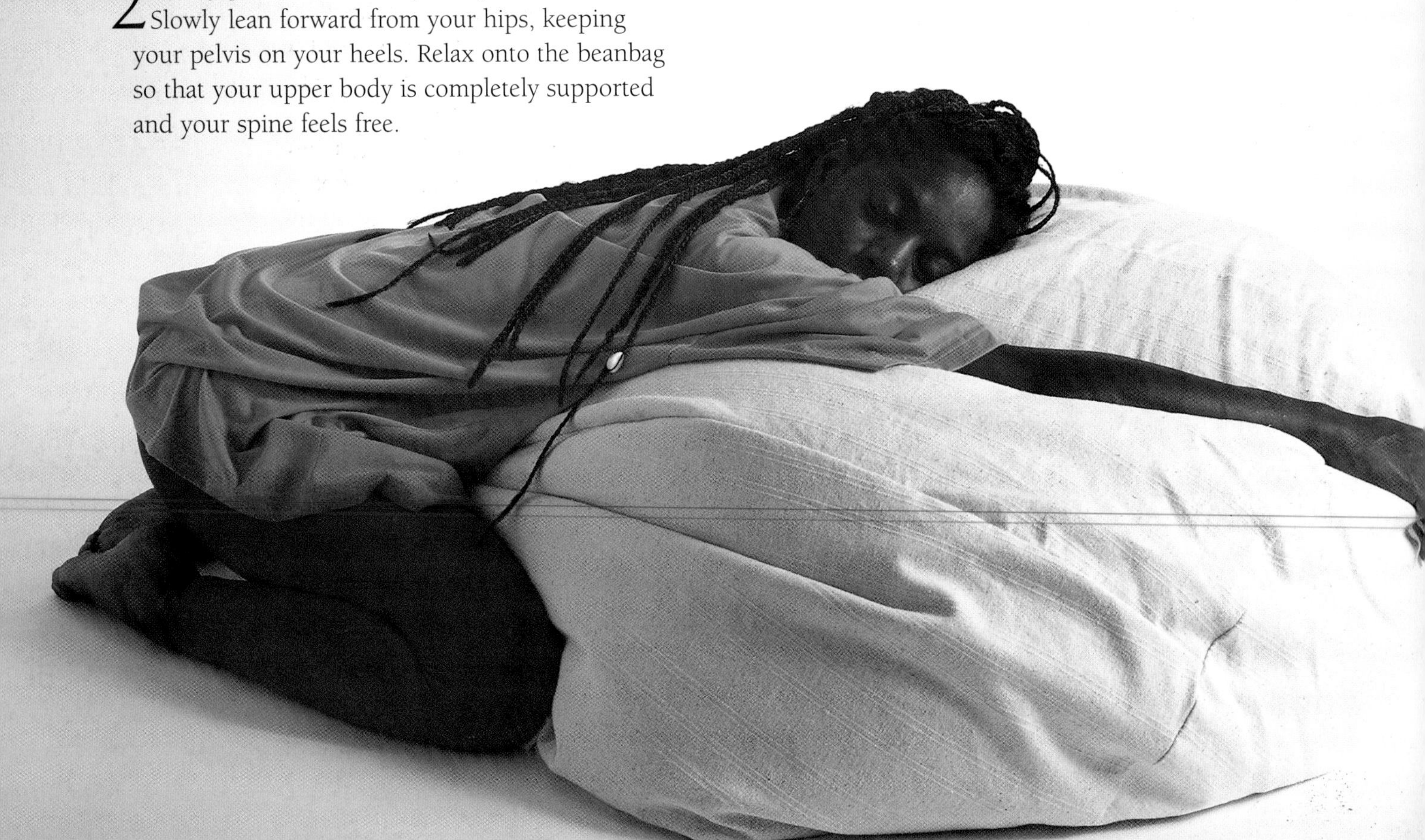

FORWARD STRETCH

This gentle stretch helps to relax your lower back and release tension in the spine, shoulders, and neck.

1 Kneel in UPRIGHT CHILD'S POSE (page 32) without using a bolster. Press the base of your spine downward and keep your pelvis on your heels throughout this exercise.

2 Slowly release your upper body forward, moving from your hips and keeping your back straight and your spine free.

3 Progress farther forward in two stages, first onto your hands as in the LEANING FORWARD exercise (page 34) and then onto your elbows.

4 Fully extend your arms out in front of you, placing your forehead on the ground or on a small cushion. Focus on the rhythm of your breathing and on the ground beneath your body.

5 Completely relax for up to one minute, breathing evenly, and then return to the upright position (see COMING UP SLOWLY, page 35).

Remember

This exercise, though not essential, can be enjoyable if you find the movement to be easy. If your back bends or if you feel any strain as you go forward, omit this exercise, and do RESTING OVER A BEANBAG opposite.

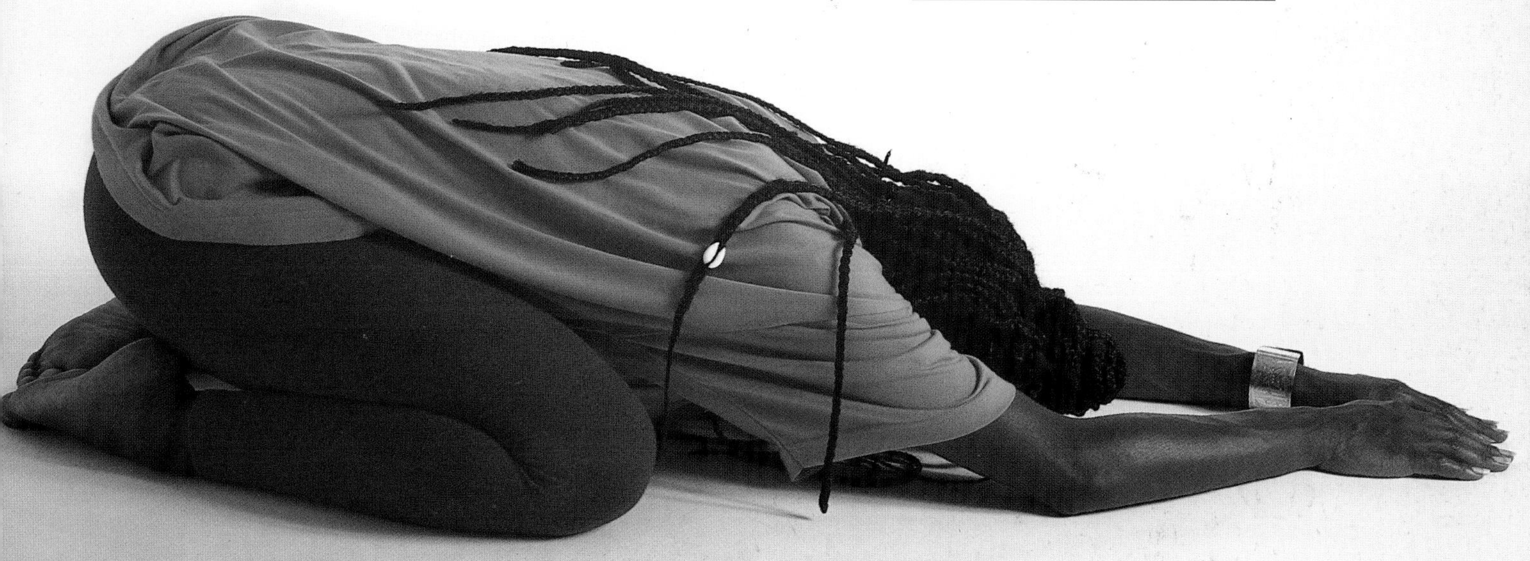

BABY HAMMOCK

This simple exercise releases tension in the lower back and prevents and eases backache. Kneeling on your hands and knees in late pregnancy encourages your baby's spine to rotate downward toward the ground with the pull of gravity, allowing the baby's back to lie in the "hammock" of your stomach muscles. This is called the anterior position and is the best way your baby can lie for labor and birth. This exercise also helps to prevent the baby from lying "posterior" (its spine against your spine) as the birth approaches.

1 Kneel down and place your palms on the floor in line with your shoulders. If your wrists are swollen or aching, rest your hands on a soft pillow. You can also do this exercise leaning forward onto the seat of a low chair, with your arms folded and supporting your weight, and your back horizontal.

2 Put your knees in line with your hands and your feet in line with your knees.

3 Relax your neck and gently let go of the weight of your head. Breathe evenly, and be aware of the way your hands and knees make contact with the floor.

HANDS, FEET, AND KNEES IN LINE

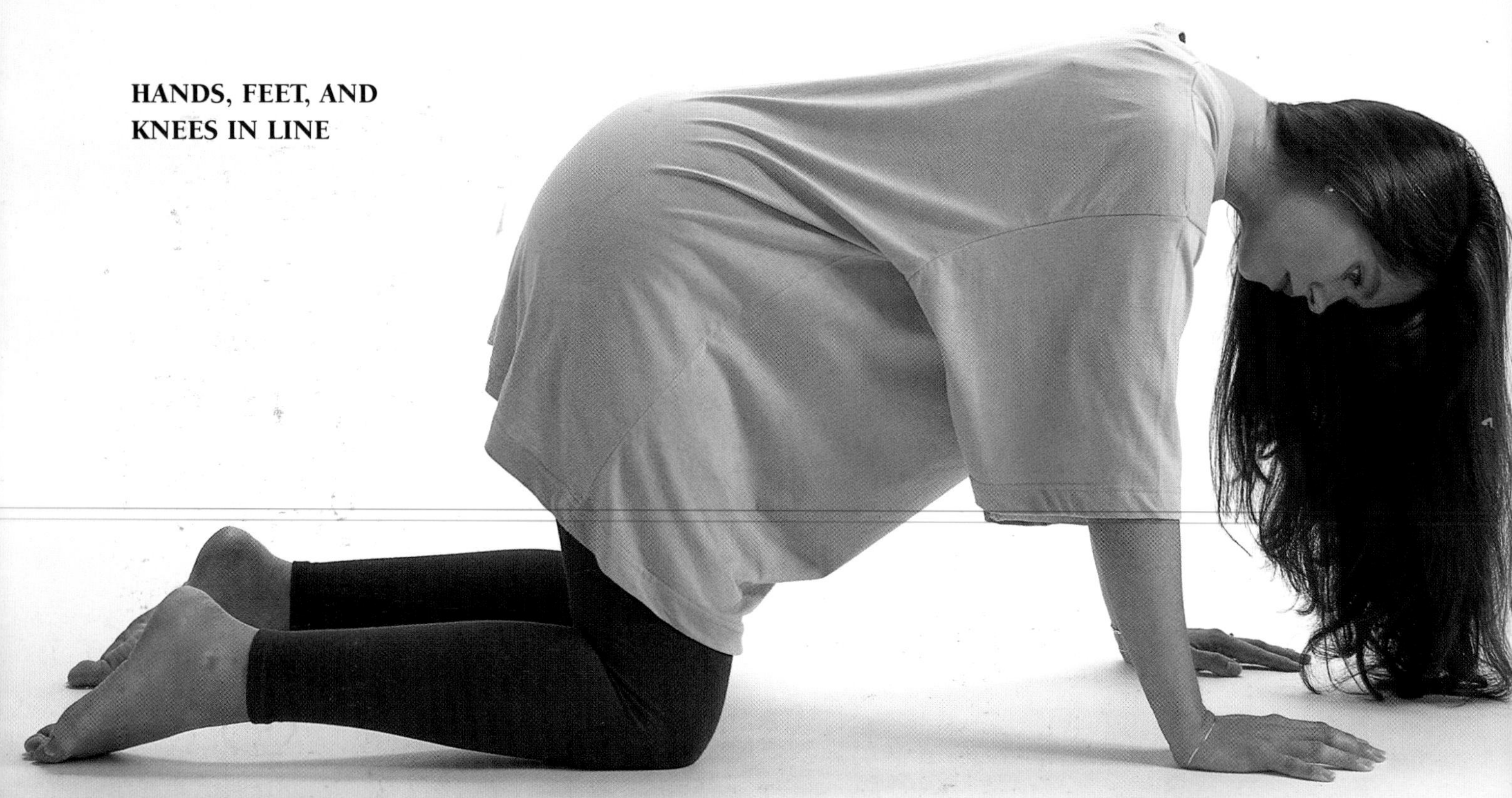

4 Breathe out slowly and lengthen the base of your spine gently downward toward your heels so that your back becomes softly rounded like a bridge—tuck your pelvis under your lower back as you lengthen your back downward.

5 At the end of the exhaled breath, gently tighten and squeeze your buttock muscles, holding for one or two seconds. Return to the starting position with your back horizontal as you inhale.

6 Repeat these movements up to ten times, moving gently with the breathing rhythm.

Remember

Make these movements gently without tensing any muscles as you tuck your pelvis under. Avoid arching or hollowing your lower back when you breathe in.

PELVIC TUCK

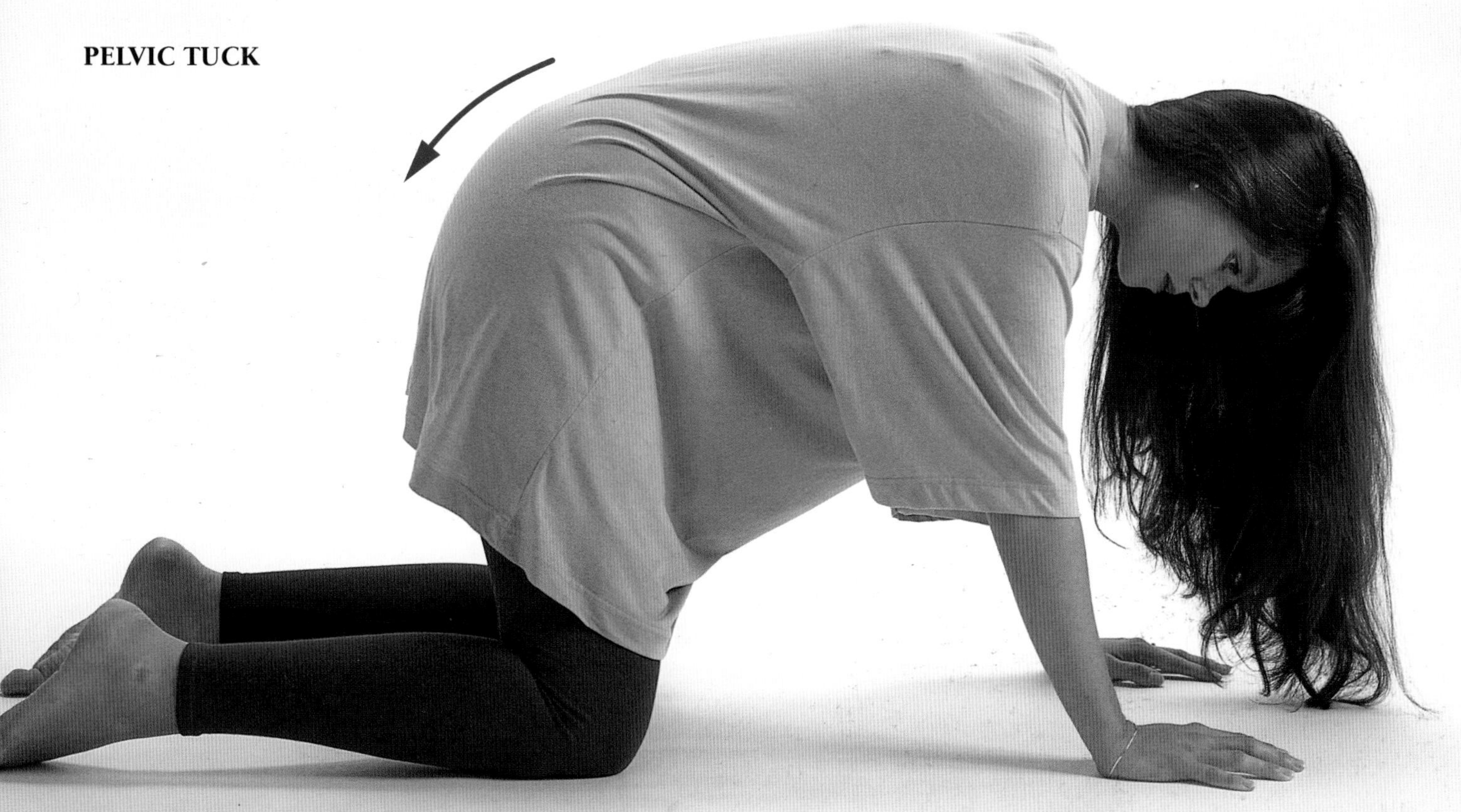

GOOD STANDING

Standing correctly is especially important in pregnancy, when the extra weight you are carrying exaggerates your spinal curve. Any imbalance can cause back pain or sciatica. Lengthening your lower back downward helps to prevent excess arching at the back of the waist—a common cause of back pain in pregnancy. Do this exercise daily, and practice it whenever you have to stand for long periods. If you feel faint after standing up for a few minutes, then omit this exercise or try it for a shorter period of time.

1 Stand with your feet about twelve inches (hips' width) apart. Your feet should be parallel and your heels should be placed slightly wider apart than your toes.

2 Lift and spread all your toes, and then relax them on the floor. Repeat this two more times. Make sure that your knees are loose and relaxed so that the energy can flow through your legs.

3 Stroke your lower back downward with your hands and, as you do so, gently ease the heavy base of your spine.

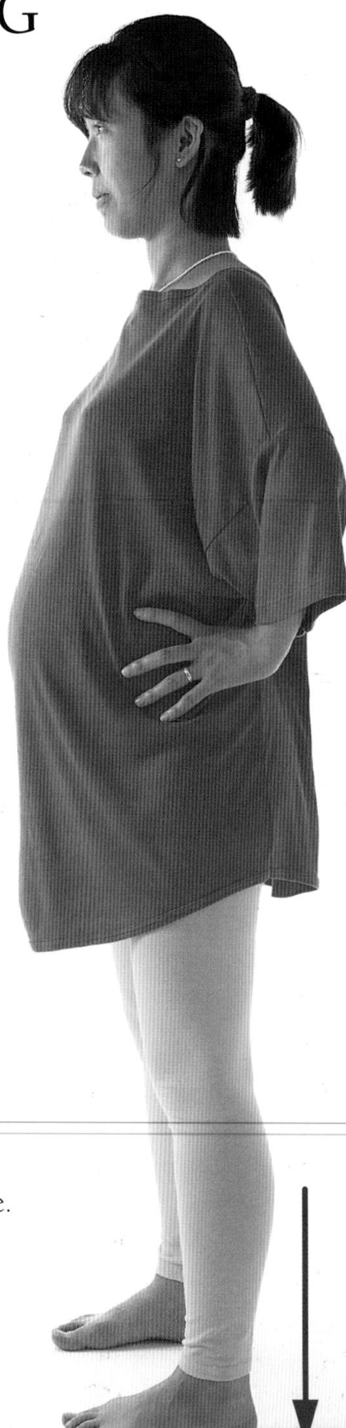

4 Place your hands on your hips for a few seconds. Relax and drop your shoulders, letting your arms hang loosely by your sides. Relax the back of your neck by slightly releasing your chin down toward your chest.

5 Breathe evenly. Notice how your body weight drops down through your lower back toward the ground, through your hips, legs, and feet. Sense how your body is weighted to the ground from the pelvis down, and lifted upward from the waist.

6 Hold for a few cycles of the breathing rhythm, moving out of the position whenever you want to.

Remember

Always keep your heels slightly wider apart than your toes and your lower back pressing downward when you stand and walk. This may feel strange at first, but once you get used to it, you will feel how spreading your heels apart releases tension in your lower back, spine, and shoulders.

BENDING FORWARD

This movement allows you to release tension in the back of your legs, to lengthen and release your spine, and relax your shoulders all at the same time. Try doing it at the kitchen counter or table while you are waiting for water to boil! However, do not do this exercise if bending forward makes you feel light-headed.

1 Face a table or counter in the GOOD STANDING start position on the opposite page. Release your lower back downward and drop your weight through your heels into the floor.

2 Keep dropping your heels, and breathe out as you slowly lower your upper body, bending from the hips. Place your palms on the table top with arms outstretched.

3 Be aware of the heavy base of your spine, and lengthen and release the rest of the spine from the waistline toward the top of your neck.

4 Hold the position for a few seconds, enjoying a feeling of relaxation and release along the spine and a gentle stretch at the back of your legs. Notice the pull of gravity through your heels now and also when coming up.

Remember

Keep your hips in line with your heels when you bend forward. Your spine should feel long and free, as you feel the stretch in the back of your legs.

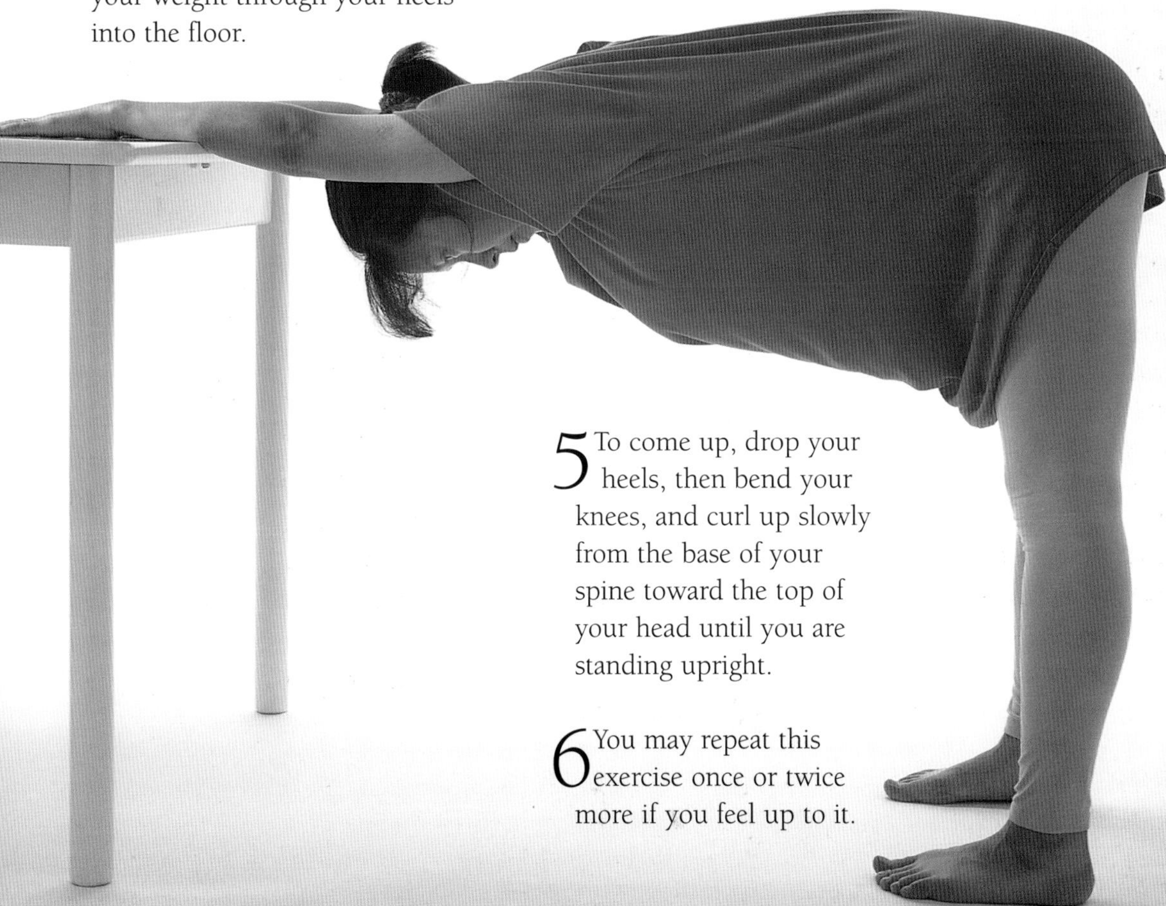

5 To come up, drop your heels, then bend your knees, and curl up slowly from the base of your spine toward the top of your head until you are standing upright.

6 You may repeat this exercise once or twice more if you feel up to it.

GENTLE STANDING TWIST

For releasing tension in the back, neck, and shoulders, and for maintaining flexibility of the spine.

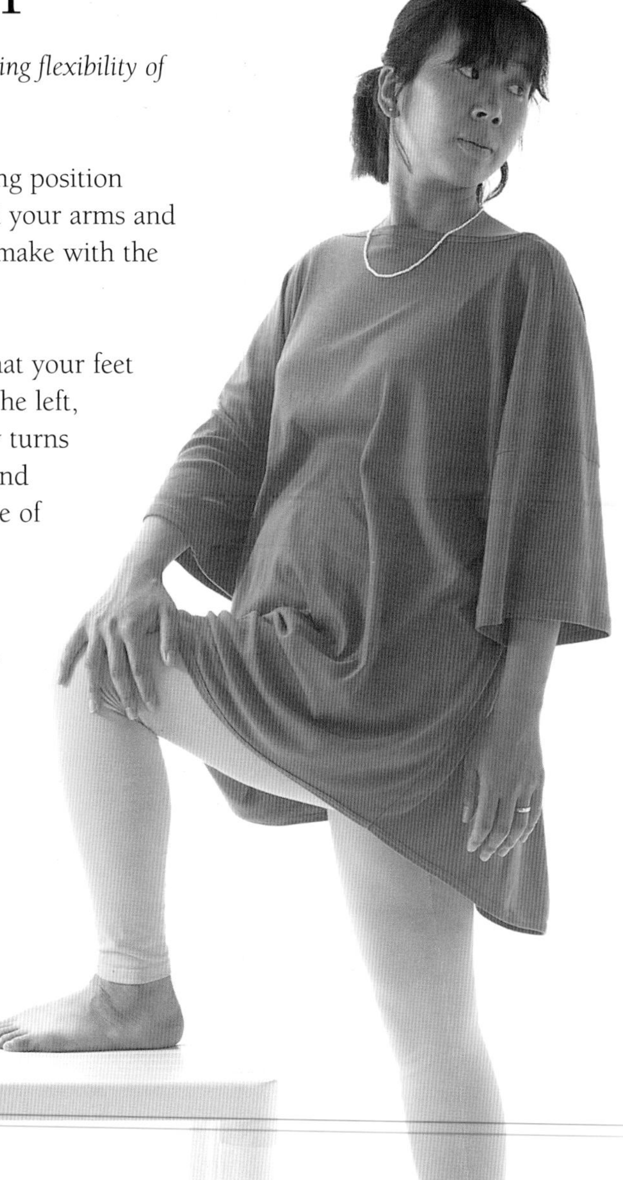

1 Place a stool in front of you. Stand in the GOOD STANDING starting position (page 40), with your lower back releasing toward the floor and your arms and shoulders relaxed. Breathe evenly and feel the contact your feet make with the floor as your weight settles into your heels.

2 Place your left foot on the stool in front of you, making sure that your feet are still parallel. Breathe, and slowly turn your upper body to the left, keeping your feet and hips facing forwards. As your spine gently turns from the base up to the top of your neck, relax both shoulders and place your right arm across your body, gently holding the far side of your bent knee.

3 Let your left arm hang loosely from your shoulder as you turn your neck and head gently to the left. Release the left shoulder down and back, and hold the position for about three to five cycles of the breathing rhythm. Slowly turn to face forward.

4 With both feet still in position, turn your body to the right, placing your right hand over your knee and gently holding the other side of your thigh.

5 Look over your right shoulder, relax the arm and release the shoulder softly back and down. Hold for three to five cycles of the breathing rhythm, and come slowly back to face forward. Return to the standing position.

6 Repeat the exercise, this time placing your right foot on the stool, turning first to the right, and then to the left. .

Remember

Turn gently without straining. Feel the contact with the ground the foot of your straight leg is making as the weight falls through your heel.

CALF STRETCH

.This exercise lengthens and relaxes the calf and hamstring muscles at the back of the legs. Regular practice will help to relieve leg cramps and also will make squatting easier.

1 Stand about twelve inches away from a wall with your feet parallel to each other. Clasp your hands, and place your forearms against the wall. Relax your neck and shoulders.

2 Put your left leg behind you, keeping your left knee straight. Simultaneously bring your right leg forward, bending your right knee. Make sure your feet are straight and that they face the wall. Your hips should be parallel to the wall, and your shoulders should be relaxed.

3 Breathe evenly and drop your left heel onto the floor. Your right foot should rest lightly on the ground as your weight falls onto your back heel. Feel the stretch in the back of your left leg as you hold this position, breathing evenly for three to five cycles of the breathing rhythm.

4 Change legs so that your left leg is forward with the knee bent and the right leg back. Breathe evenly. Hold the position for three to five cycles of the breathing rhythm and then change legs. Repeat the exercise once more on each side and then return to the GOOD STANDING position (page 40).

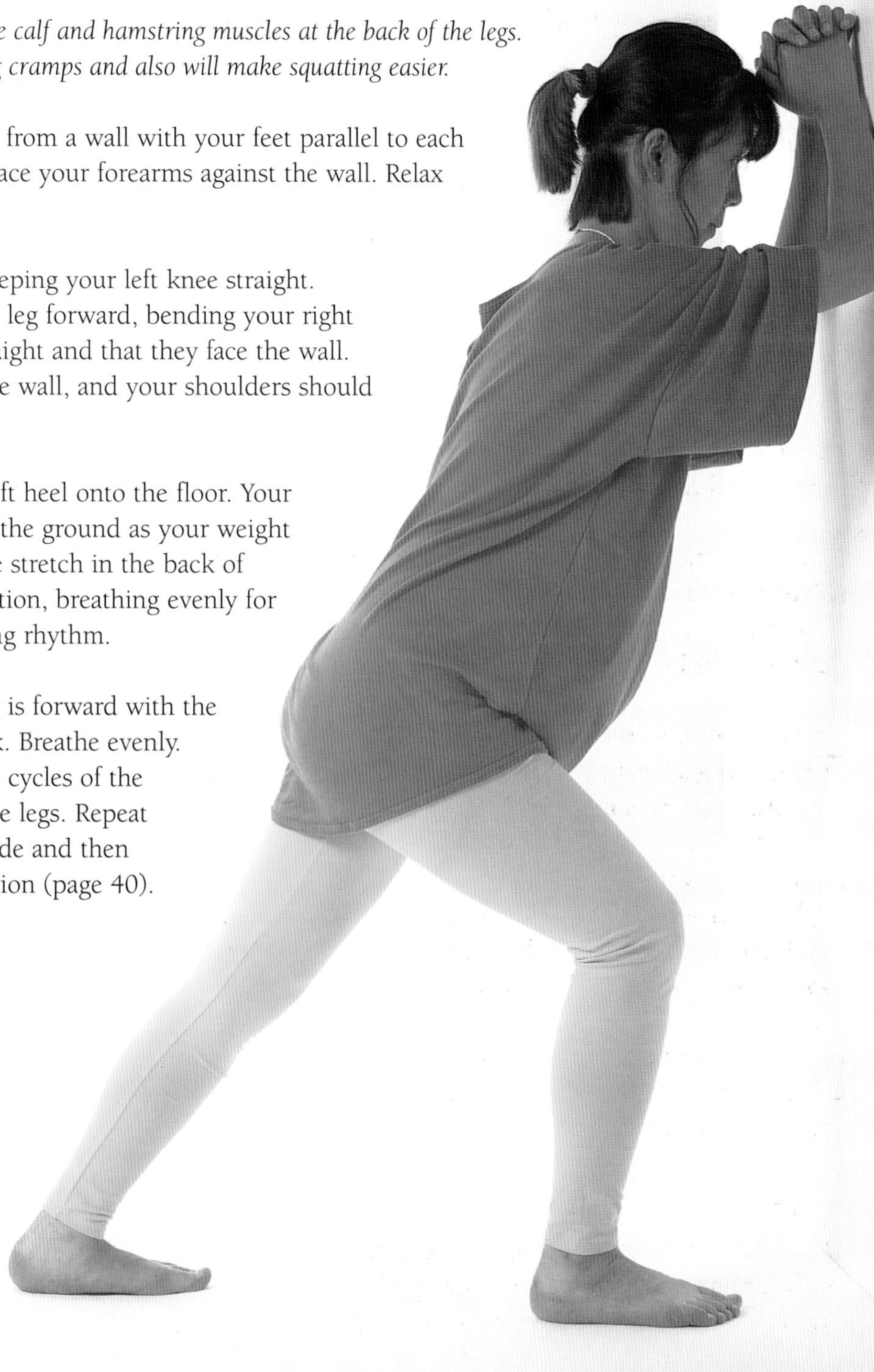

SQUATTING

USING A STOOL

Squatting in pregnancy helps to improve flexibility of the pelvic joints and to gently increase the diameters of the pelvis. Squatting on a stool as you do in this exercise will encourage your baby's head to engage in late pregnancy. Use this position instead of a full squat during the last six weeks of pregnancy or if you find squatting to be difficult.

1 Put a small cushion on a low stool or on a ten-inch high pile of heavy books, and position it against a wall. Stand with your feet a little wider apart than in the GOOD STANDING position (page 40) and slightly turn them out.

2 Feel the way your feet make contact with the floor. Breathe evenly, releasing your weight down through your heels into the ground.

3 As you breathe out, slightly bend your knees, keeping your heels on the floor.

4 Slowly continue this movement until your pelvis drops down gently into a squatting position, with your buttocks resting on the stool and your knees spread apart in line with your feet.

5 Lengthen your spine against the surface of the wall.

6 Remain in this position for up to five minutes, and then come up slowly.

Remember

Using a stool reduces pressure on the cervix and pelvic floor, so use this position only during the last six weeks of pregnancy, avoiding those shown on pages 45–47; avoid them altogether if you have vulvitis, hemorrhoids, full or partial placenta previa, or a cervical suture (stitch).

HOLDING ON

This supported squat is slightly more challenging than the previous one and can be practiced through the first 34 weeks of pregnancy. If you find it too difficult or uncomfortable, use a stool. Otherwise, it is a good idea to alternate between using a stool and holding on to a support when you practice.

Remember

Keep your spine long and avoid bending your back when you squat. Do not do this exercise during the last six weeks of pregnancy.

1 Stand facing a firm support, such as the edge of a table, a window ledge, or the side of a bathtub. Place your feet apart as you did in the previous exercise, and breathe evenly, putting your weight onto your heels.

2 Hold on to the support, and, keeping your heels down and your arms straight, bend your knees and slowly lower your pelvis into a squat. Your knees should be spread comfortably wide apart, with your feet mimicking the angle of your knees.

3 Breathe evenly and hold the position for about three cycles of the breathing rhythm.

4 Drop your heels back and come up slowly as you breathe out.

5 Repeat this exercise two or three times.

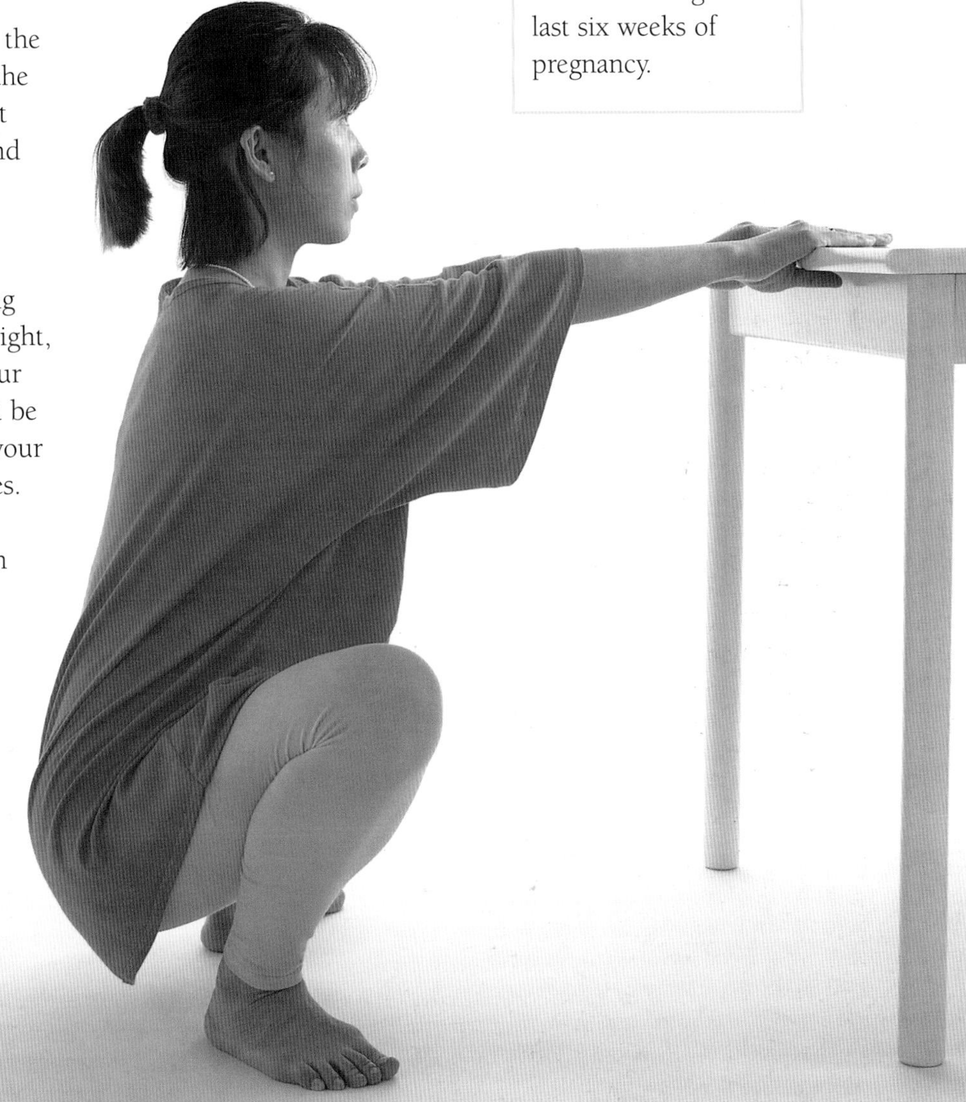

FULL SQUAT

Do this exercise only if you feel completely at ease in the USING A STOOL *or* HOLDING ON *exercises* (pages 44–45). *This exercise can be practiced through the first 34 weeks of pregnancy. Supporting the heels makes squatting easier for some women, but you should not do this exercise if you are not completely comfortable.*

USING A ROLL

Roll up an exercise mat or a thin blanket and place it on the floor. Stand with your feet apart as in the USING A STOOL exercise (page 44). Place the roll under your heels, and stand with your feet apart and slightly turned out.

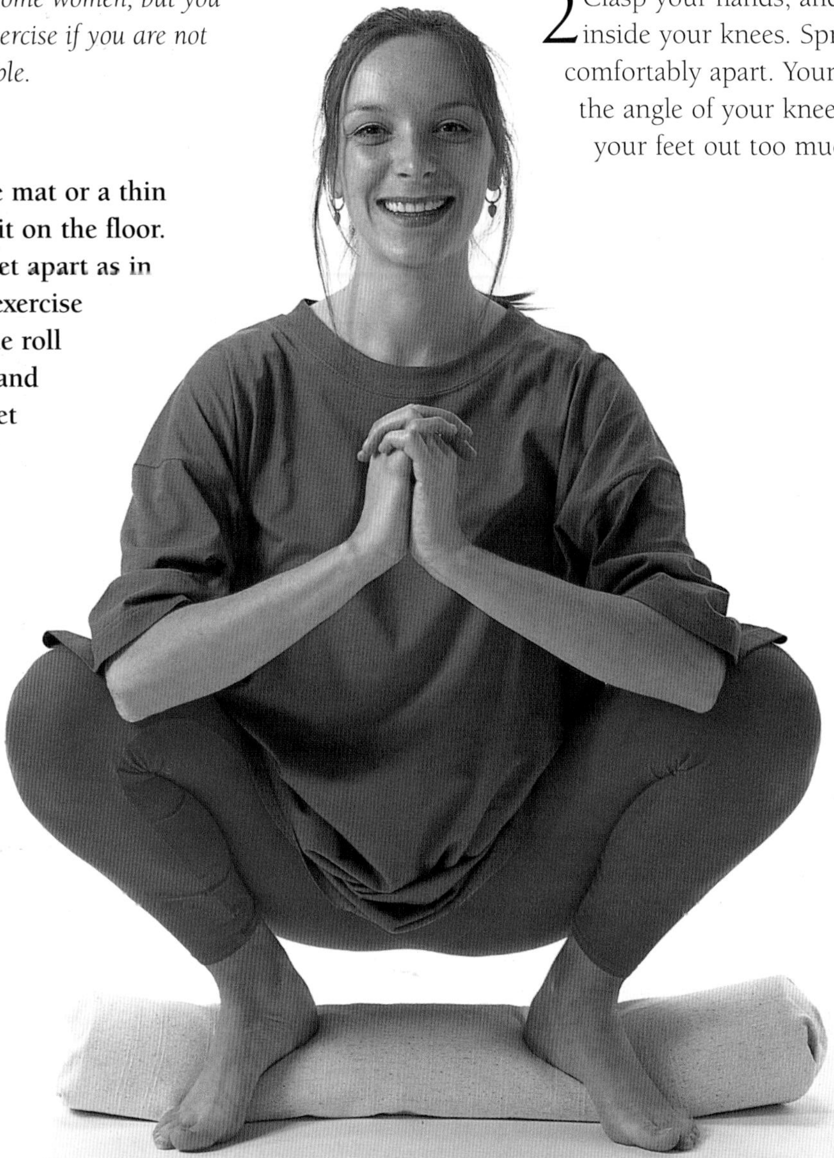

1 Slowly move down into a squat, bending your knees and lowering your pelvis as your weight falls onto your heels.

2 Clasp your hands, and place your elbows inside your knees. Spread your knees comfortably apart. Your feet should follow the angle of your knees. Avoid turning your feet out too much.

3 Lengthen your spine, leaning forward slightly from your hips if it feels comfortable.

4 Breathe evenly and hold for three to five cycles of the breathing rhythm.

5 Move up slowly, dropping your weight into your heels, or roll forward on your hands and knees and then rise.

WITHOUT SUPPORT

Stand as you did before with your feet apart and slightly turned out. Drop your heels and breathe evenly. Use this position only if you can do it easily or comfortably.

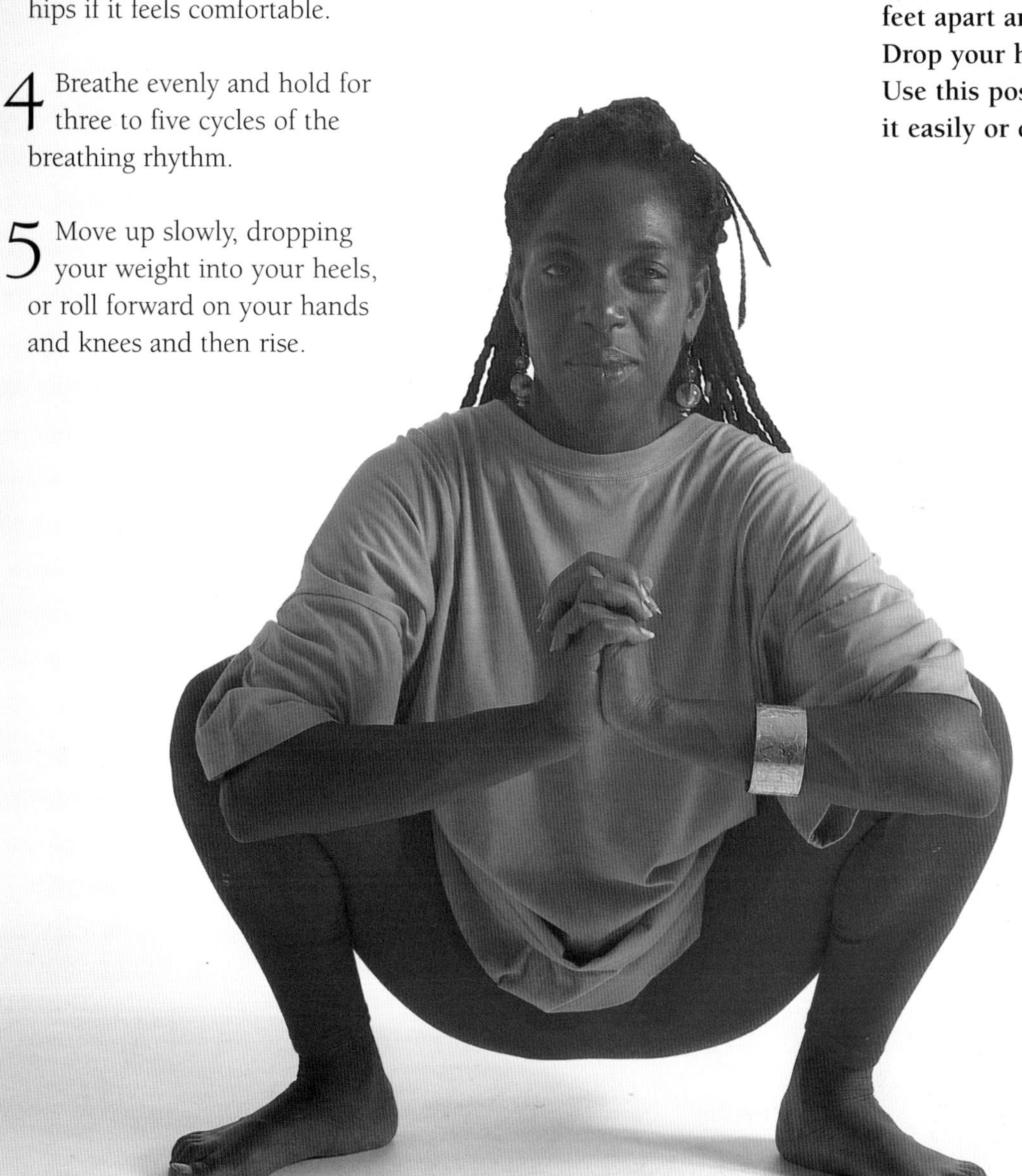

Remember

Keep your spine long, and avoid bending your back. In the last six weeks of pregnancy, it is best to use a stool and to keep your spine against a wall when you squat (see page 44). This will help your baby's head to engage.

THE PELVIC FLOOR

Strengthening your pelvic floor will help you while you are pregnant and during and after the birth. There are two special pelvic exercises that you can practice regularly, QUICKIES (pages 50–51) and THE ELEVATOR (pages 52–53), and four positions in which you can do them. Before you try them out you should understand where your pelvic floor is, how it functions, and why these exercises are so important.

What is the pelvic floor ?

Inside the base of your pelvis, there is a layer of muscle shaped somewhat like a hammock which forms the floor of your pelvis. It extends across the bottom of the pelvis, from the pubic bone in front to the tailbone at the back, and also from side to side, from one hipbone to the other. The muscle fibers of the pelvic floor are arranged in three interconnecting rings, or sphincters, around the openings to the pelvic organs: in front in the urethra (leading to the bladder); in the center in the vagina (leading to the uterus); and at the back in the anus (leading to the bowel).

The function of the pelvic floor

The pelvic floor supports the weight of your pelvic and abdominal organs and the weight of your baby while you are pregnant. The muscles also control the opening and closing of your bladder and bowel. Your baby's head and body will pass through the center of the pelvic floor when you give birth. The muscle fibers soften and relax in pregnancy to allow this to happen more easily. After the birth, they regain their strength and tone.

The benefits of exercising the pelvic floor

Pelvic floor exercises involve both tightening and contracting movements as well as releasing and letting go, and have two important benefits:

1 The tightening or contracting movements improve muscle tone and strengthen the pelvic floor. This ensures that there is good support for the increasing weight of the pelvic and abdominal organs in pregnancy. Good muscle tone will also maintain control of the opening and closing of the bladder and bowel and improve or prevent such problems as incontinence, vulvitis, and hemorrhoids. These problems arise when the muscle tone of the pelvic floor is too loose. Problems tend to be more common in pregnancy, when these muscles become softer in preparation for the birth. Regularly doing pelvic floor exercises while you are pregnant reduces the risk of damage to the pelvic floor during childbirth and also results in good muscle tone and a quick recovery after the birth.

2 The relaxing and releasing movements help to prevent or ease constipation. Learning to focus on letting go of tension in the pelvic floor, as you

do when you release your pelvic floor muscles, also prepares you for giving birth when you will instinctively release and relax these muscles as your baby's head and body emerge.

How to tell whether you are using the right muscles

1 Next time you empty your bladder, try stopping the flow in midstream. The muscles you will be contracting are your pelvic floor muscles. Then try tightening the same muscles after your bladder has emptied.

2 When you are in the bath, insert one finger in your vagina and tighten the muscles inside to grip your finger. These are your pelvic floor muscles. When you tighten or contract these muscles you will find that the front, center, and back of your pelvic floor all move in unison.

Don't worry if your buttock or stomach muscles move as well—with practice you will learn to move your pelvic floor muscles on their own.

Positions for pelvic floor exercises

Pelvic floor exercises can be done in four different positions—**all fours**, **knee chest**, **half squat,** and **easy squat**—shown below and on pages 50–53. You can choose any one of them for both exercises and vary your choice each time you practice or change your position midway.

If you have hemorrhoids or vulvitis in pregnancy, regular practice of these exercises will help to improve or eliminate discomfort. However, do them only in the **all fours** or **knee chest** positions on pages 50–51, and omit the squatting positions.

How often should I do pelvic floor exercises?

Once you have chosen the position that you find to be most comfortable, do both THE ELEVATOR and QUICKIES in succession. These exercises should be done at least three times a week. QUICKIES can be done on their own at any time and in any place, as often as you like, but once a day is plenty.

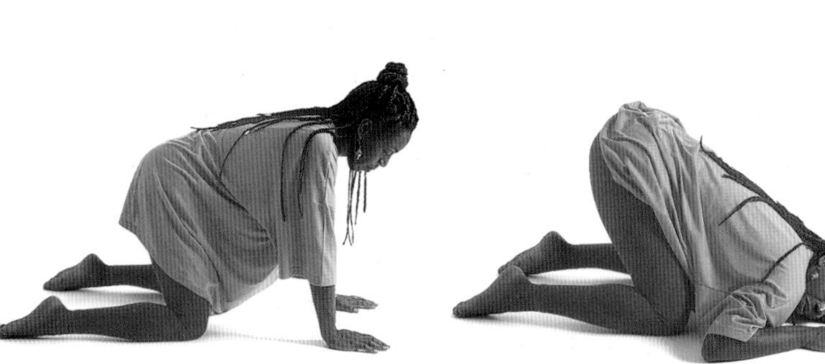

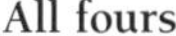

All fours

Knee chest

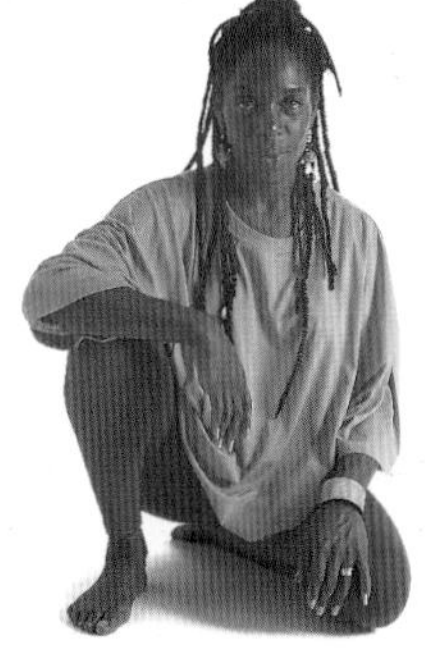

Half squat

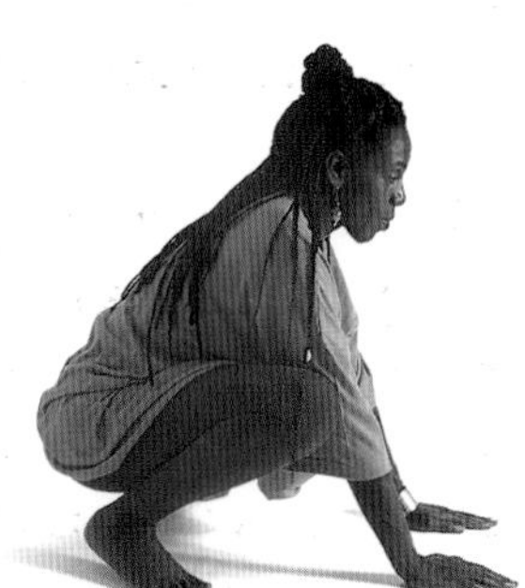

Easy squat

QUICKIES

Quickies encourage good muscle tone of the pelvic floor and can be done on a daily basis. Do them in any of the positions shown on pages 50–53. You can continue doing these after giving birth to strengthen your pelvic floor and aid your postnatal recovery.

1 Choose one of the four positions from this page and the following three pages and make yourself comfortable, breathing in your normal rhythm.

2 Focus on your pelvic floor and tighten the muscles, pulling them up inside.

ALL FOURS

Kneel on your hands and knees, placing them about twelve inches apart, with your back flat like a table. Spread your palms and your fingers, and make sure your feet are in line with your knees. Lower your head, and relax your neck and shoulders. Feel the ground underneath you as you breathe comfortably.

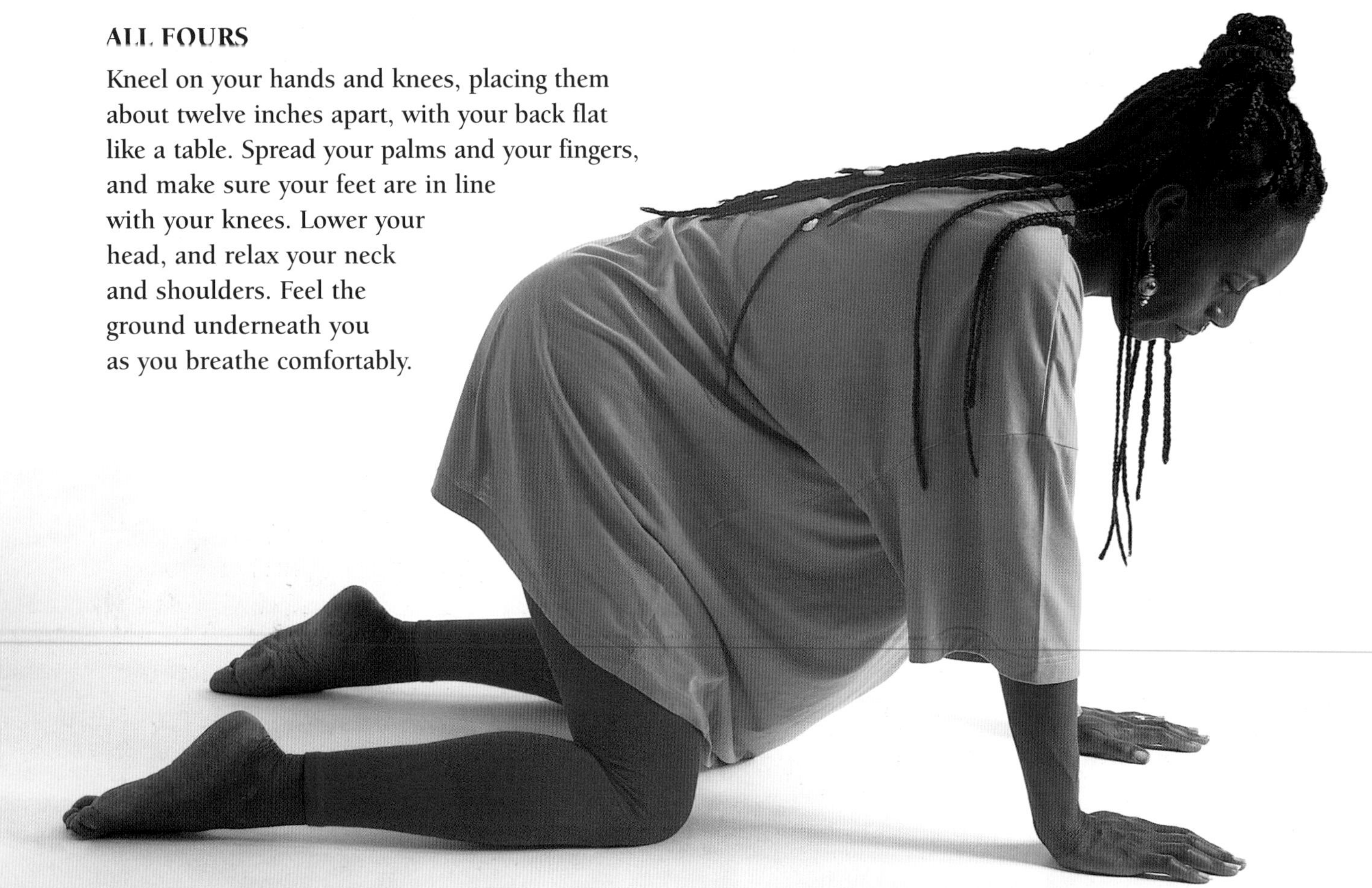

3 Hold for five seconds, and then slowly let go.

4 Repeat the first two steps ten times, and then stop.

5 Relax for a few moments and then repeat this exercise two more times.

KNEE CHEST

Start in the all fours position on the opposite page. Lean forward from your hips, and place your lower arms on the ground. Turn your head, and rest your face on the ground. Relax your neck and shoulders. Focus on the floor underneath you and the flow of your breathing.

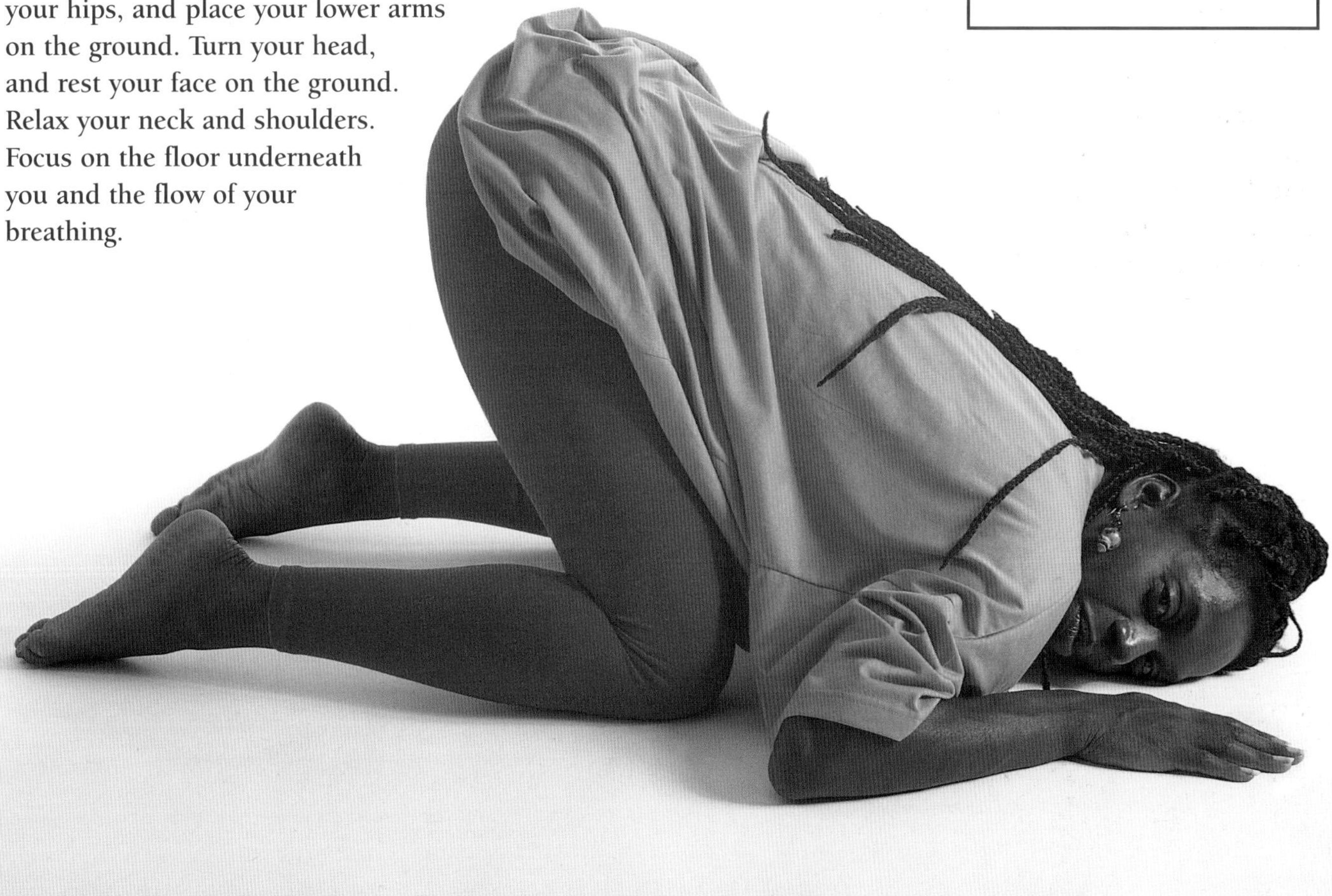

Remember

To relieve the discomfort of hemorrhoids or vulvitis, try doing 50–100 quickies in the knee chest position first thing every morning and last thing every night. Continue in this manner each day until there is a marked improvement, and then reduce this number to 25–50 QUICKIES twice a day.

THE ELEVATOR

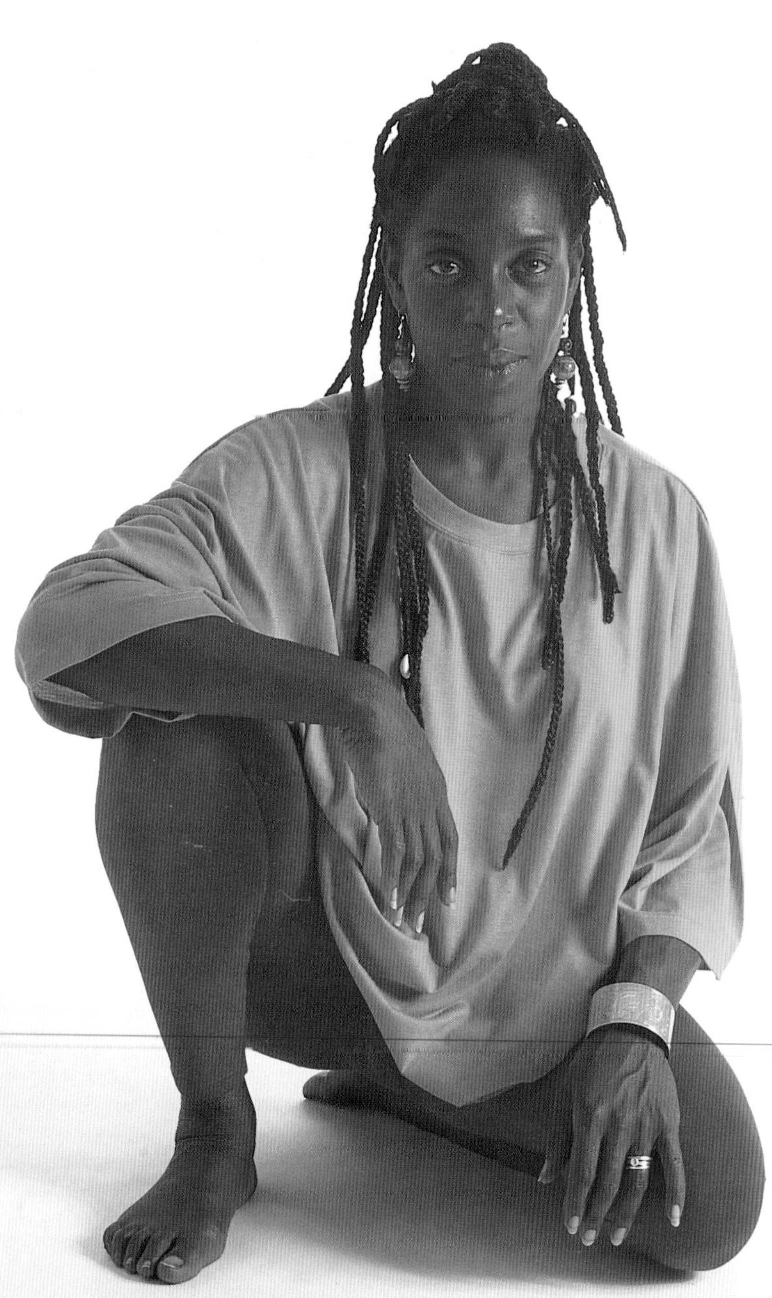

To gradually tighten your pelvic muscles, imagine an elevator in a four-story building as you do this exercise. You will begin in the "basement" and then go up to the "fourth floor." Pause briefly at each "level" on the way up and as you go back down.

1 Make yourself comfortable in one of the four pelvic floor exercise positions.

2 Breathe in your normal rhythm. Close your eyes, and focus on your pelvic floor.

3 Start in the "basement" and contract your pelvic floor muscles, slightly drawing them up toward your uterus and pausing on the "first floor."

4 Tighten them a little more until you reach the "second floor", and pause. Repeat in this way until you get to the "third" and "fourth floor".

HALF SQUAT

Kneel on the floor and sit back on your heels. Bend one leg and place the foot flat on the floor. Position your arms and legs so that they are comfortable, and relax your neck and shoulders. Be aware of the floor beneath you and of the rhythm of your breathing.

5 Breathe normally while you hold tight the pelvic floor muscles on the "top floor" for a second or two.

6 Gently release your pelvic floor muscles in stages as you descend, "floor" by "floor." Pause at each level for one second on the way down.

7 Relax the pelvic floor completely as you descend to the "basement." Rest for a moment, and repeat the exercise twice.

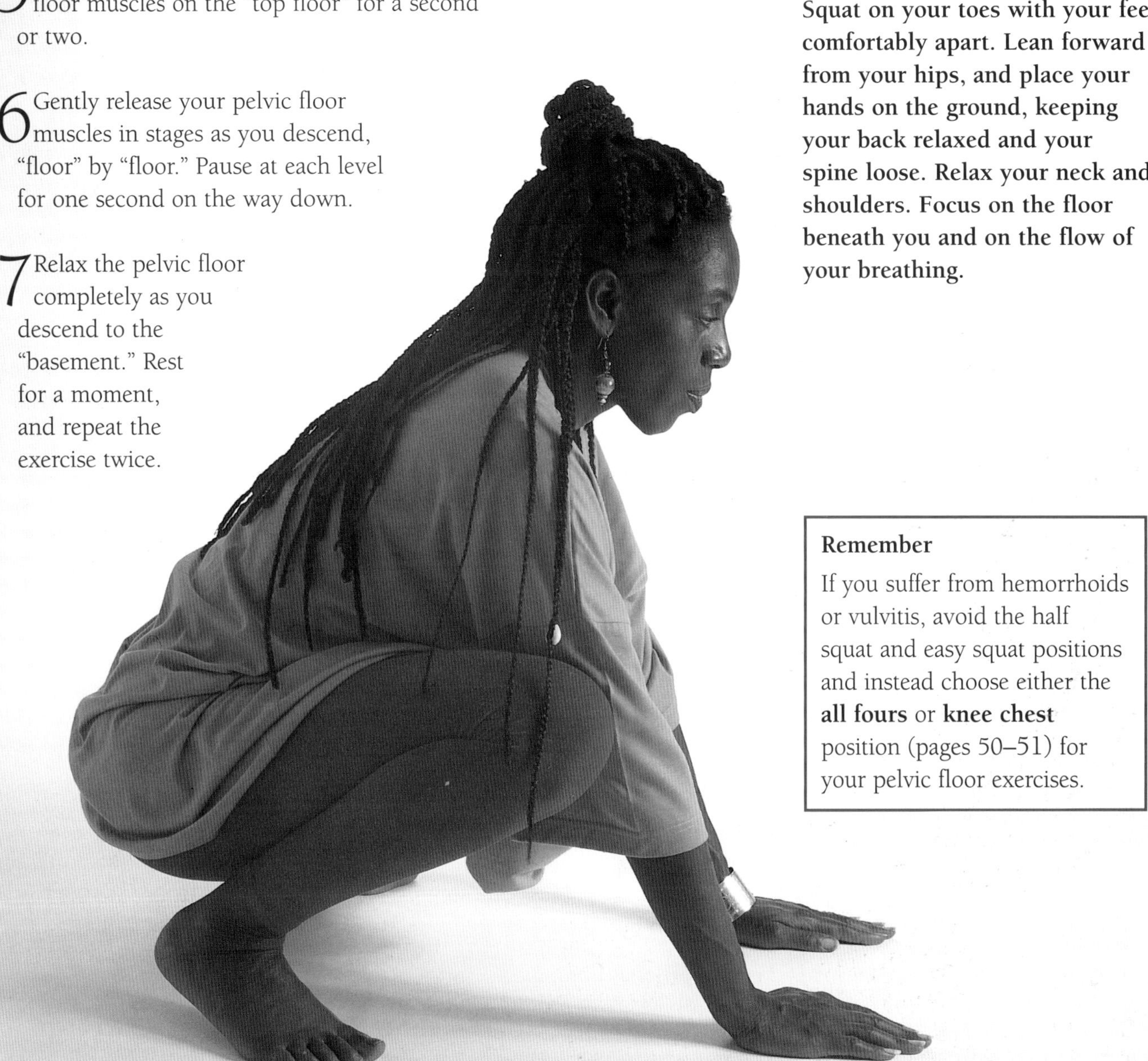

EASY SQUAT

Squat on your toes with your feet comfortably apart. Lean forward from your hips, and place your hands on the ground, keeping your back relaxed and your spine loose. Relax your neck and shoulders. Focus on the floor beneath you and on the flow of your breathing.

Remember

If you suffer from hemorrhoids or vulvitis, avoid the half squat and easy squat positions and instead choose either the **all fours** or **knee chest** position (pages 50–51) for your pelvic floor exercises.

PREPARATION FOR LABOR

It is a good idea to prepare for labor throughout your pregnancy. If you practice the movements on page 57–61, they will soon become comfortable and familiar body habits, and it will be easy and natural to use them later on in labor. You will also be encouraging your baby into a good position for birth and helping your baby's head to engage in the rim of your pelvis.

The last weeks of your pregnancy are special. You need to rest more and focus on preparing mentally and physically for birth. This will enable you to approach the experience well rested and relaxed. Try to spend an hour or so each day doing your favorite exercises, including BREATHING and BABY AWARENESS (pages 12–13), the RELAXATION positions on pages 62–65, and the exercises in this section.

Going into labor

Labor will start when your pregnancy reaches full term and your baby is ready to be born. This can happen any time between the 37th and 43rd week of pregnancy, although the average length is 40–41 weeks. You may experience a "pre-labor" in which mild contractions may last several hours or even overnight, and then stop. This is very common and prepares your body for labor.

The exercises presented thus far have been preparing you to work through the contractions you will experience during labor. You have been learning how to focus awareness on your breathing, how to be in contact with the ground beneath you, and how to relax your body and release tension while you exercise. This is all great practice for staying relaxed during labor and for coping with the power and intensity of the contractions. After a while you will get used to the rhythm of working though the contractions and resting in between them. Usually, pain increases toward the peak of each contraction and then gradually fades away. The resting phases between contractions are pain free and give you a chance to relax and replenish your energy. It is a continual rhythm of work and rest, allowing your body to surrender as your uterus slowly opens to allow your baby to be born.

While the contractions themselves are intense and are likely to be painful at the peak, the peaceful rests in between make it possible to go along with this rhythmic process. A contraction lasts about thirty seconds in early labor and builds up to a minute or so by the time you are almost ready to give birth.

Think of your labor positively, as a personal birth dance. After all, you are helping your baby to be born. Express yourself freely with your body and respond with movements to the pain, exploring which movements make you most comfortable. These will also be the best movements to help your baby on his or her way through the birth canal.

You may find the easy upright positions and movements on the following pages helpful to use when you are in labor.

Upright positions

Very few women, if left to their own instincts, would choose to lie on their backs or in a semi-reclining position in labor. This is a custom that developed in the Western world along with a more medical approach to birth. However, today it is becoming widely recognized that when mothers can move freely in labor and choose their own comfortable positions, there are many benefits to both mother and baby:

- Upright positions are more comfortable and reduce pain, helping the mother to be more in control of her labor.
- Contractions are more effective, resulting in a shorter labor.
- The blood supply to the baby is improved, reducing the risk of fetal distress.
- The baby's journey through the pelvis is easier because the diameter of the pelvis is wider in an upright position, and the downward force of gravity helps the baby to descend.

Using upright positions increases your chances of an uncomplicated birth and makes it less likely that you will need medical intervention. However, if you do need help or choose some medication, you will probably find that the techniques you have learned from your exercises will help you. You can approach the experience from a position of power and feel good about it in the end, as well as make a rapid recovery afterward.

How to practice for labor

For the exercises on pages 57–61, you will need a chair, a pillow, a low stool, and a beanbag or a pile of large cushions. When you practice these movements, imagine that you are experiencing a real contraction in labor using a combination of position, movement, and breathing to get through it. Think of the contraction like a wave in the ocean. It begins gently and gradually, builds up in intensity to reach a peak, and then begins to decline until it's gone.

Choose one of the positions, and then move your body freely in that position as you focus on your breathing. Practice breathing throughout the wave of the contraction, concentrating on breathing out through your mouth and then inhaling slowly through your nose. There will be three to five cycles of the breathing rhythm per contraction.

Start as soon as the imaginary contraction

begins, focusing on breathing out and "breathing pain away" through the peak of the contraction until it subsides. Then rest and relax for a while, using one of the resting positions suggested at the end of each exercise. Let go of your body and your mind completely when you are resting so that every muscle is relaxed. Breathe in your normal rhythm, in and out through your nose while resting. As the contractions get stronger you may find that you need to make more noise as you exhale through your mouth. This will help you to release and let go of the pain. Step 3 of "Breathing awareness for labor" (see next column) includes exercises involving breathing with sounds to help you prepare for this. You should also stay grounded while in the middle of a contraction (see step 2).

In the weeks approaching the birth, practice for labor every day for five to ten minutes, combining position, movements, and breathing. On the day your labor actually occurs, wait as long as possible until you are in established labor before you use the labor positions. When the contractions become so strong that you can focus only on them—that's when you begin to work with these positions.

There are three simple breathing exercises you can try in each of the labor positions shown on pages 57–61. Try moving your body freely as you imagine breathing through a contraction in labor. Afterwards, choose one of the recommended resting positions.

Breathing awareness for labor

1 Slowly exhale through your mouth so that you can hear the sound of the exhaled breath. Pause at the end of each exhalation and inhale slowly through your nose. Continue for three to five cycles of the breathing rythm, and then relax.

2 Repeat step 1, this time focusing on the contact your body is making with the ground. Direct the exhalations downward as if to breathe the pain away into the ground each time you breathe out, and then breathe in slowly. Again, continue for three to five cycles of the breathing rhythm. Then relax.

3 This time, repeat step 2, but make some low vowel sounds as you exhale. Try "ooh" and "aah," releasing the sound from deep inside. Many women find that expressing sounds freely in labor helps to reduce pain. Continue with three to five cycles of the breathing rhythm, and relax.

STANDING

Standing up and moving during contractions helps to encourage the progress of labor. Leaning forward as you move will ease the pain and position your baby well. Relax in one of the resting position referred to below in between contractions.

1 Stand with your feet well grounded and comfortably apart so that your whole body feels loose and relaxed.

2 Hold onto the back of a chair and bend your knees. Roll your hips slowly, making gentle circular movements, or swing your hips slowly from side to side.

3 Work through a practice "contraction" (see BREATHING AWARENESS on the opposite page), and then relax in a resting position.

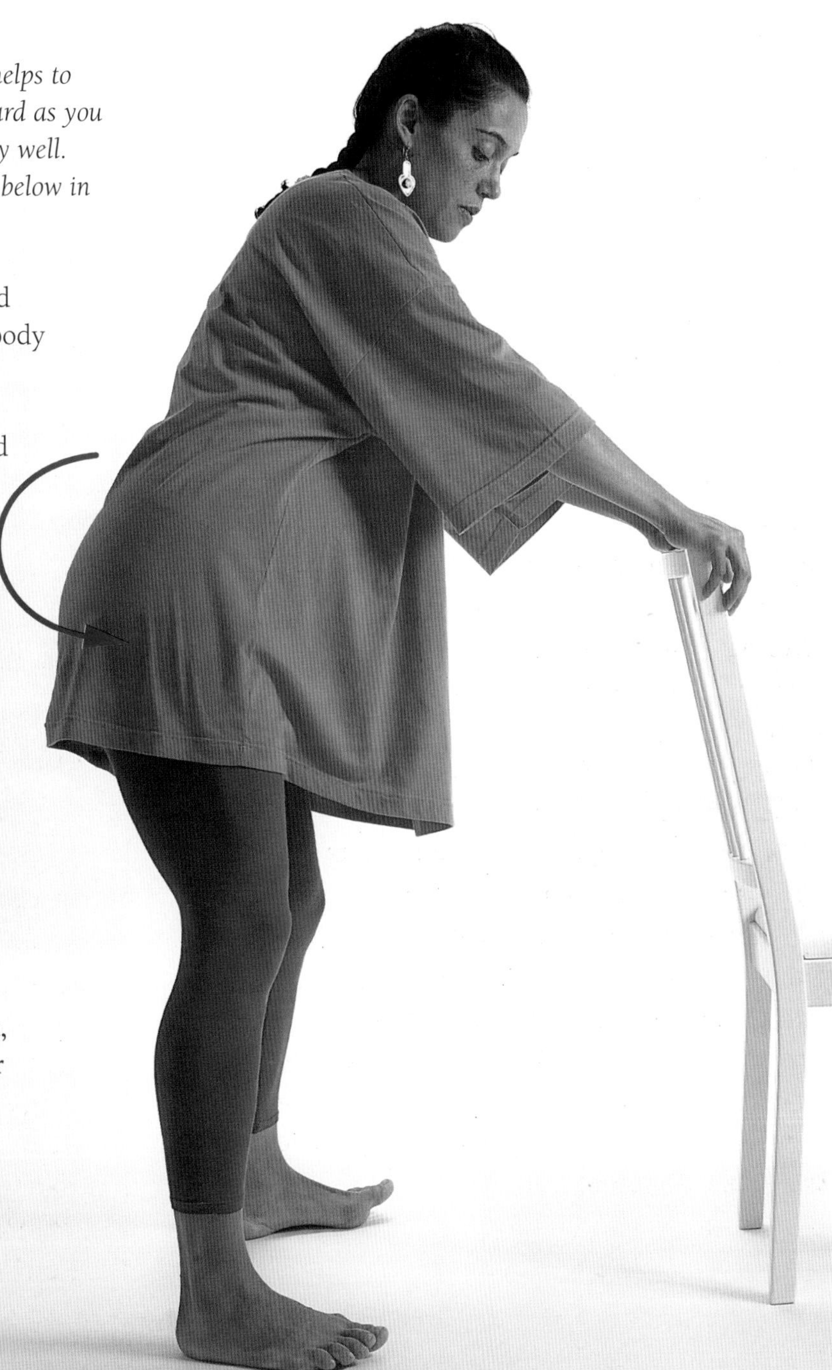

RESTING POSITIONS

- **Do some easy supported squatting on a stool (see page 44).**
- **Sit on a chair, keeping your knees apart, leaning forward, and resting your upper body on a support (see page 62).**
- **Sit facing backward on a chair, resting your head on a pillow placed on the back of the chair.**

KNEELING UPRIGHT

In this vertical kneeling position, gravity will help to make your contractions more effective. Use it in labor as an alternative to standing if you still have quite a long way to go. This position can also be used in a birthing pool.

1 Kneel on the floor on a soft surface with your knees slightly apart. Relax your arms and shoulders, and either rest your hands on your hips, letting them hang loosely by your sides, or hold onto a support.

2 Roll your hips, making slow, circular movements, or alternatively, swing your hips from side to side.

3 Breathe through a few practice contractions, using the BREATHING AWARENESS exercises on page 56, and then relax in a resting position.

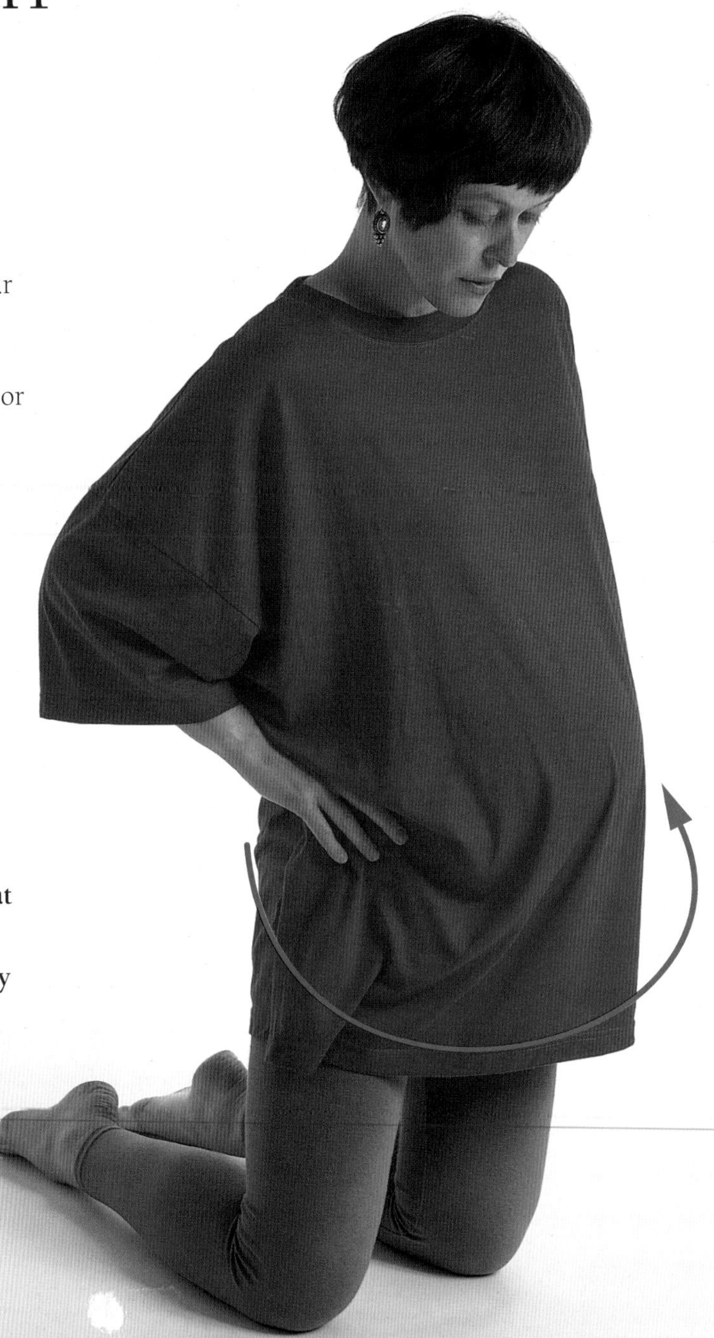

RESTING POSITIONS

- **Lean forward onto a pillow placed on the seat of a chair.**
- **Relax over a beanbag so that your upper body is completely supported (see page 63).**

Remember

You may spend a long time kneeling in labor, so protect your knees by kneeling on soft pillows or a foam mat.

HALF KNEEL/HALF SQUAT

It may be helpful to use this from time to time during labor as a variation on the kneeling positions. Many women enjoy this position and find that it helps to relieve pain.

1 Begin in the kneeling upright position on the opposite page, using a soft surface to protect your knees. Put one leg in front of you, bending the knee and keeping your foot on the floor.

2 Relax your shoulders and arms, placing your hands on your bent knee.

3 Breathing out, gently lunge forward toward the bent knee.

4 Breathing in, slowly return to the upright starting position.

5 Repeat this movement four or five times, and then change legs and repeat on the other side. Relax in a resting position.

RESTING POSITIONS

- **Kneel forward onto a beanbag (see page 63).**
- **Squat supported by a stool, leaning forward.**

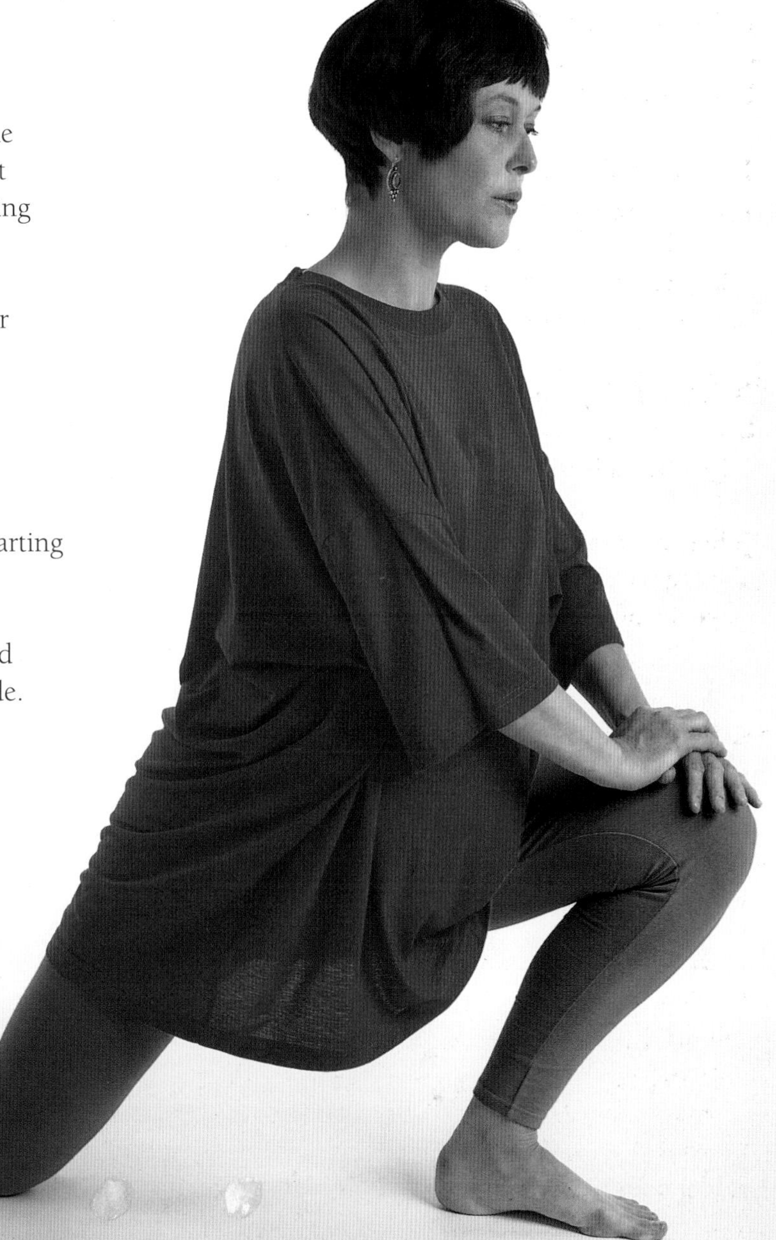

KNEELING ON ALL FOURS

Kneeling on all fours is a very secure position, offering you a lot of support and a feeling of privacy, and helping you to avoid distractions and focus on the contractions.

This more horizontal kneeling will help you to stay in control during the very fast and intense contractions that occur toward the end of your labor. This is a useful position if you have a "backache labor," and it will encourage a baby in the posterior position to turn into the more favorable anterior position by the time you are ready to give birth.

1 Kneel on a soft surface on the ground, placing your palms down and in line with your knees. You can increase your comfort during labor by placing a small cushion under each ankle.

2 Relax your neck and shoulders, letting go of the weight of your head. Breathe evenly and notice the way your hands and knees contact the floor.

3 Roll your hips, making slow circular movements, or swing your hips from side to side.

4 Practice the BREATHING AWARENESS exercises on page 56 while moving in this position, and then relax.

RESTING POSITION

From the kneeling position, lean forward onto a beanbag or a pile of large cushions (see page 63) so that your whole body is supported.

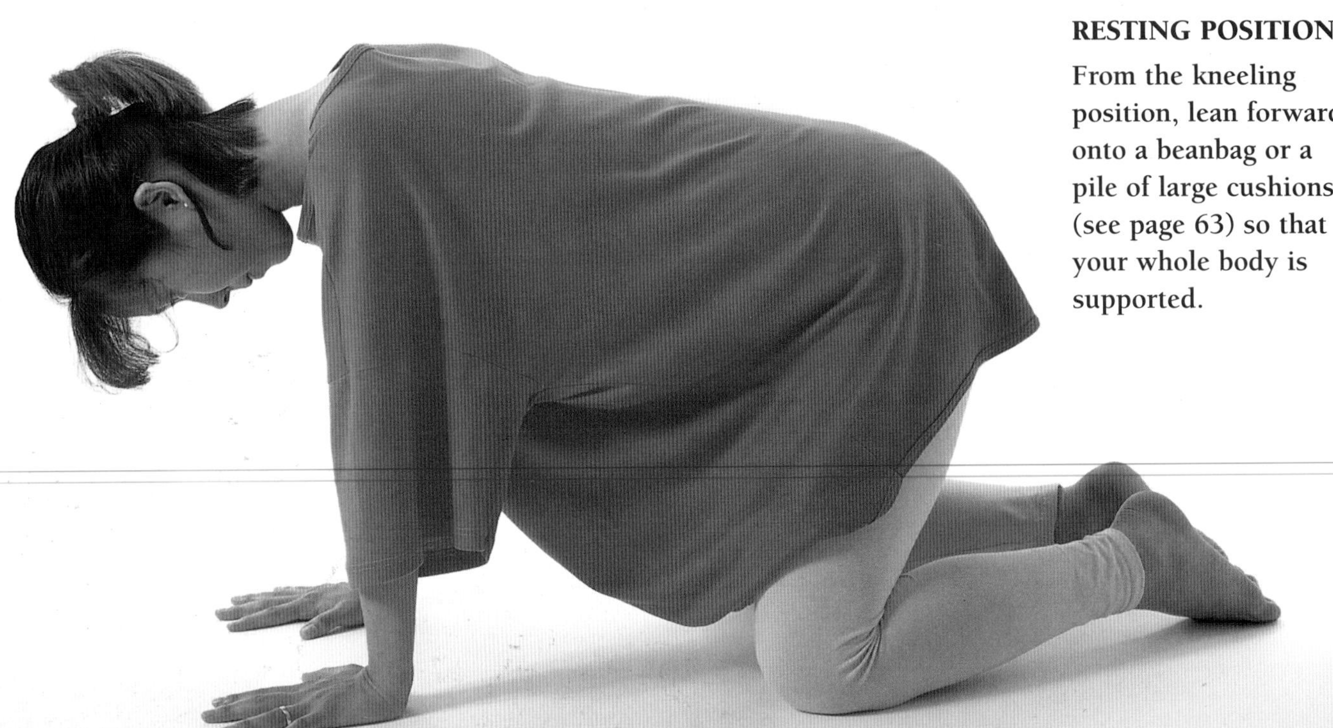

ROCKING

When kneeling on all fours in labor, it can be helpful to rock your body forward and backward and to push into the ground with your hands as a gentle form of resistance. Move slowly, and avoid arching your lower back when you come forward.

1 On a soft surface on the floor, kneel on your hands and knees. Your knees should be comfortably apart. Focus on your breathing and on the contact your body is making with the floor.

2 As you inhale, bring your weight forward onto your hands without arching your back.

3 As you exhale, bring your pelvis back toward your heels.

4 Repeat these movements five or six times, moving forward as you inhale and back as you exhale. Relax in the resting position.

5 Now try these movements using the BREATHING AWARENESS exercises on page 56.

RESTING POSITION

Kneel forward over a beanbag (see page 63) or onto a support.

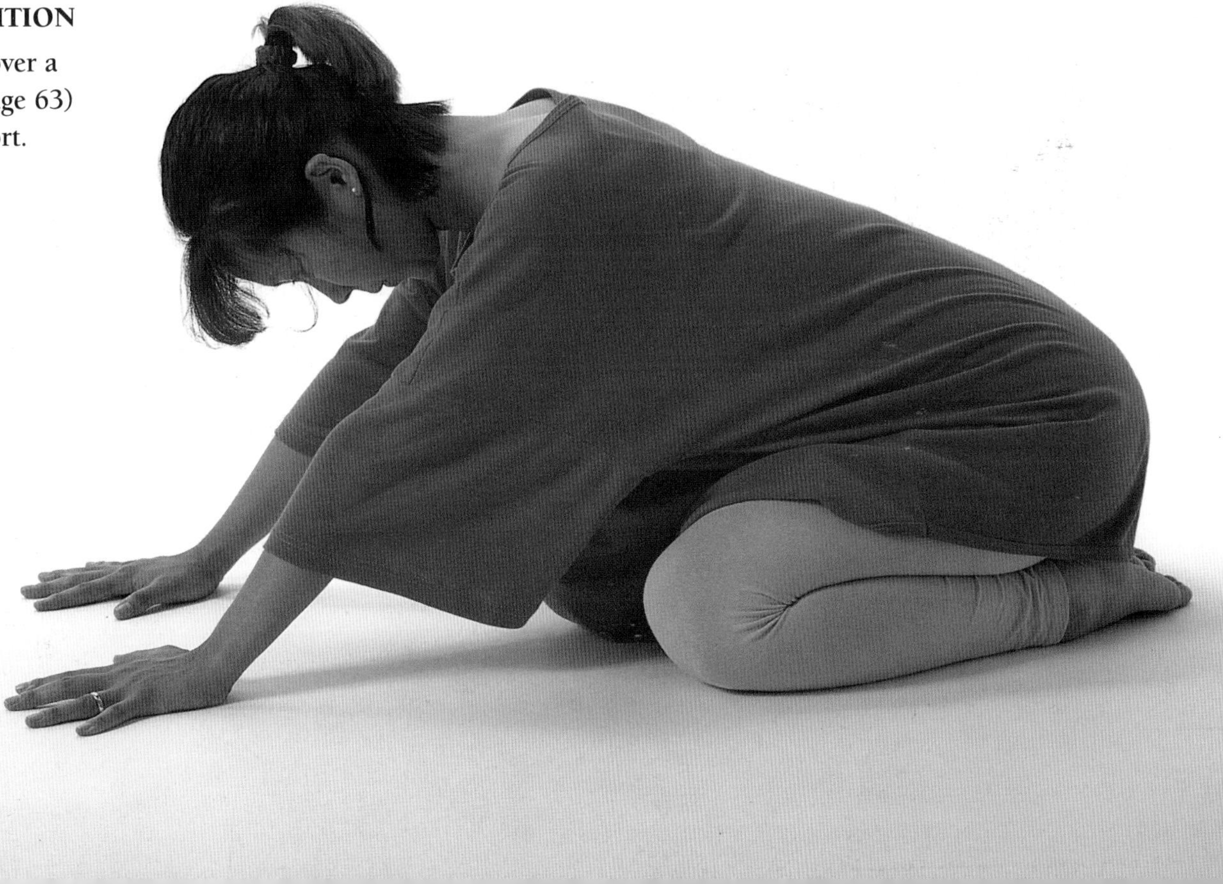

AT A DESK

Your body works hard to provide nourishment to your growing baby and to sustain and carry the increasing weight. Relaxation is very important, and you will find that you need to rest several times a day to avoid fatigue. Choose any one of the positions on pages 62–65, and remain in it for five minutes or longer, depending on how much spare time you have. Use this position to take a rest while you are working at a desk.

1 Sit on a chair with your knees spread comfortably apart and your feet flat on the floor. Place a cushion or support under your feet if necessary.

2 Lean forward from your hips onto a table or desk, with your head resting on your folded arms or on a cushion or pillow.

3 Relax your neck and shoulders, release your lower back toward the chair, and breathe evenly.

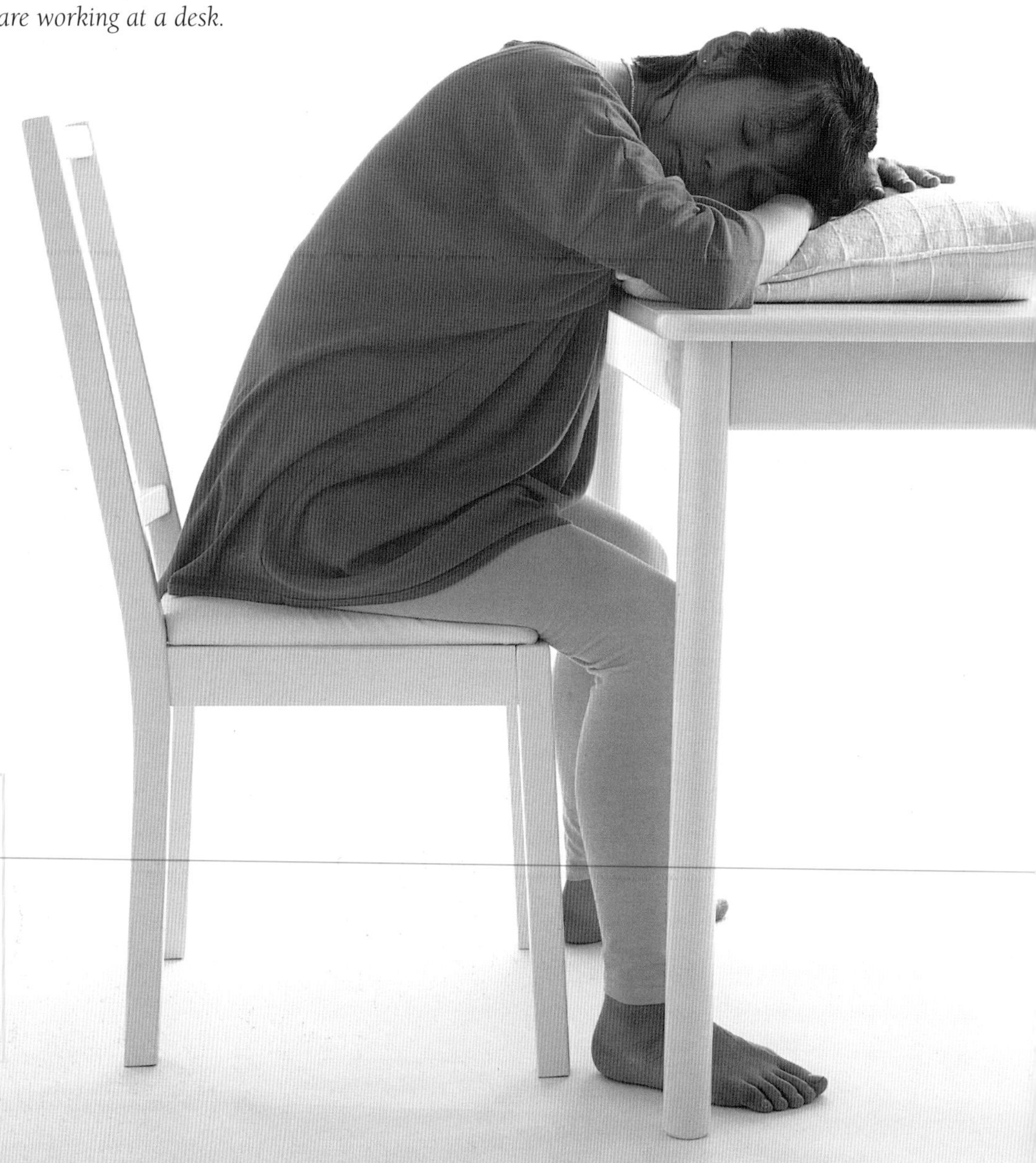

Remember

Five to ten minutes of relaxation is very helpful during a busy day. If you can, try to arrange to rest for at least half an hour after lunch.

OVER A BEANBAG

This is a wonderful resting position because it moves the weight of your baby forward, away from your lower back. It helps maneuver your baby into a good position for birth, and can be used for massage and as a resting position in labor.

1 Facing a beanbag, kneel on a soft surface on the floor with your knees apart. You can place a cushion or two between your buttocks and your calves for extra comfort.

2 Slowly move forward from your hips, keeping your pelvis down on your heels, until your upper body rests comfortably over a beanbag or several large cushions.

3 Make yourself very comfortable, molding the beanbag to fit your body, until you feel totally supported.

4 Spread your shoulders wide, rest your head, and relax your arms on the beanbag.

Remember

If you feel any discomfort in your knees, calves, or ankles, place cushions under your buttocks until your pelvis is higher than your knees, or kneel with a bolster cushion between your legs.

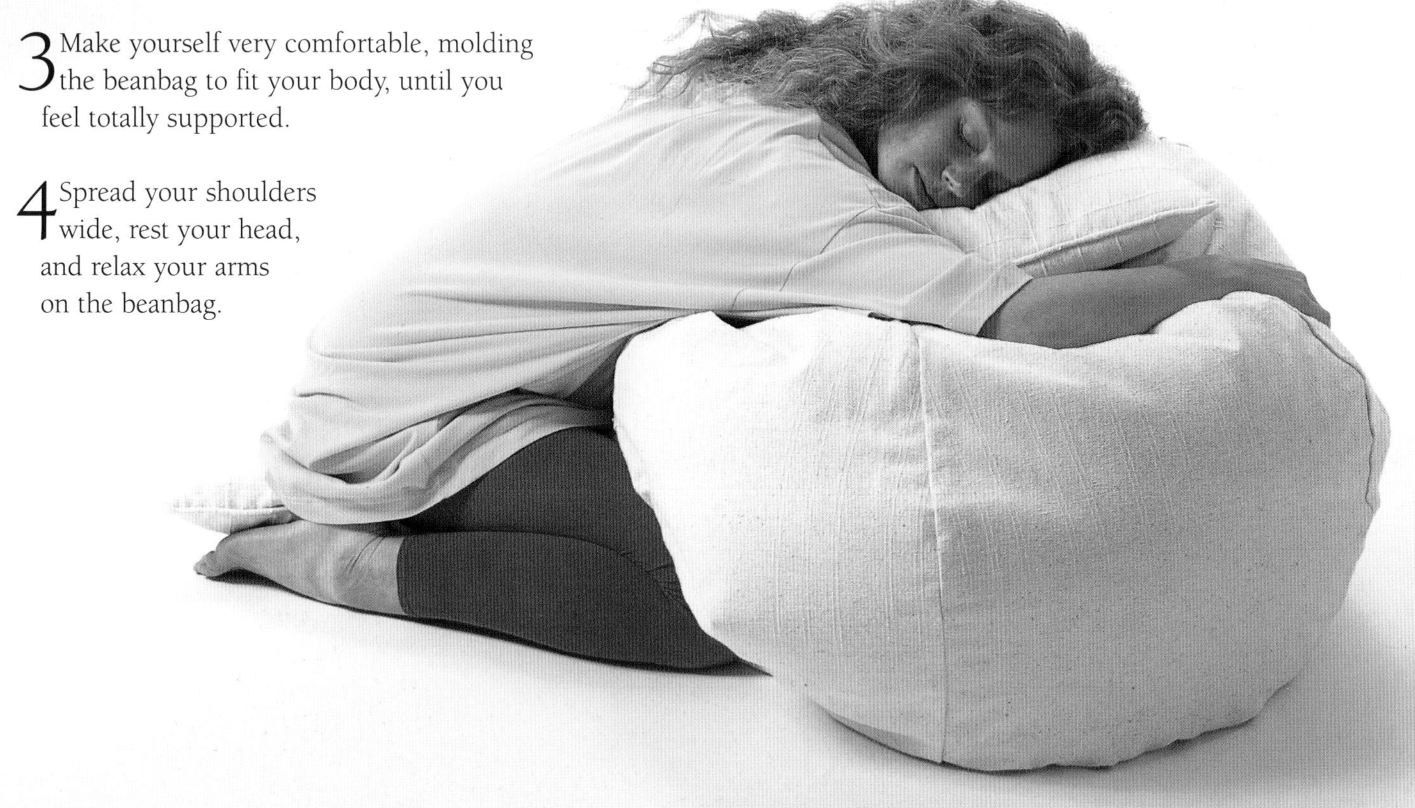

LYING ON YOUR SIDE

While some women find this position very comfortable, others prefer the FRONT SIDE POSITION *on the opposite page. Lying on your left side helps to encourage your baby's spine to the left side of your abdomen, which is the best position for labor. You may wish to vary this by sometimes lying on the right, but it is good to lie on the left when you rest and sleep, especially during the last six weeks of your pregnancy.*

1 Lie on your left side on a soft surface, with your head resting on a cushion. Extend your left leg out behind you and bend your right leg, placing a pillow or two under your right knee.

2 Make sure that your arms are positioned comfortably, that your neck and shoulders are relaxed, and that you can breathe easily.

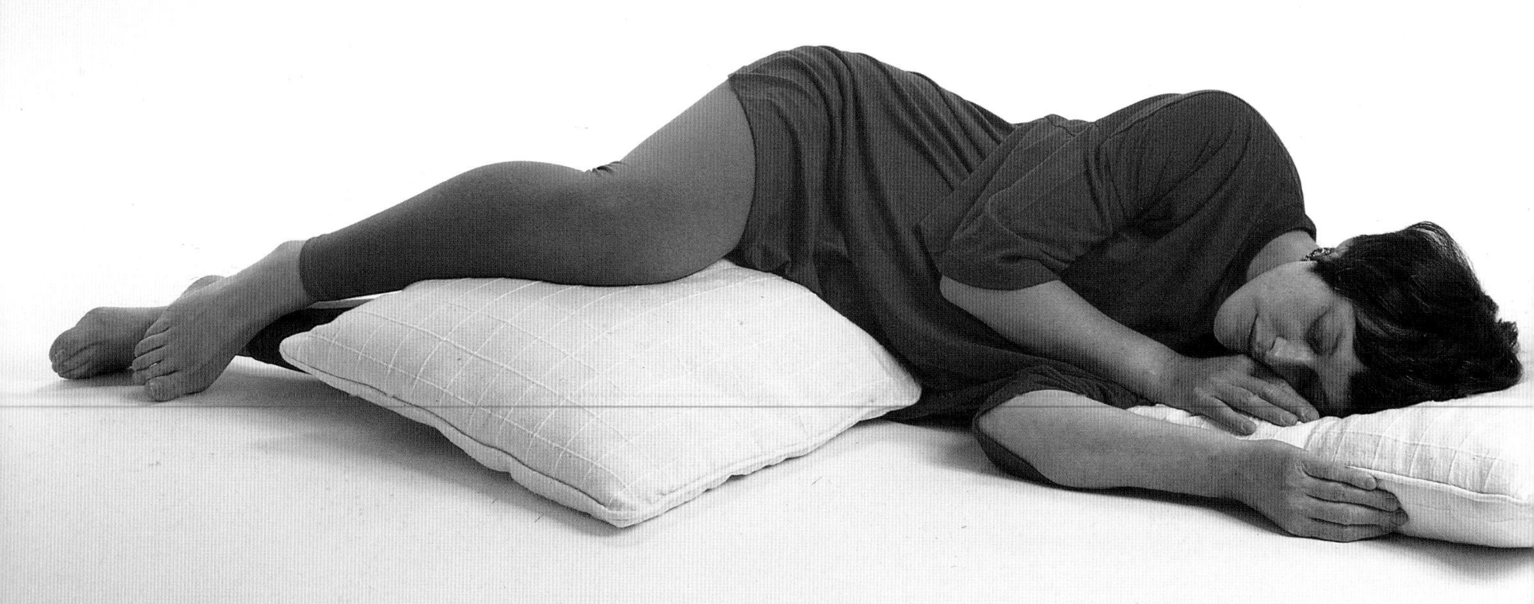

FRONT SIDE POSITION

1 Lie on your left side on a soft surface, with your head resting on a cushion. Extend your left leg out behind you and bend the right one, placing a pillow or two under your right knee for comfort.

2 With your upper body facing the ground as if you were lying on your front, extend your left arm downward behind you and your right arm upward in front, with your shoulders spread out and relaxed.

3 On a small cushion, rest your head so that it's facing your right hand. Make sure that you feel completely comfortable.

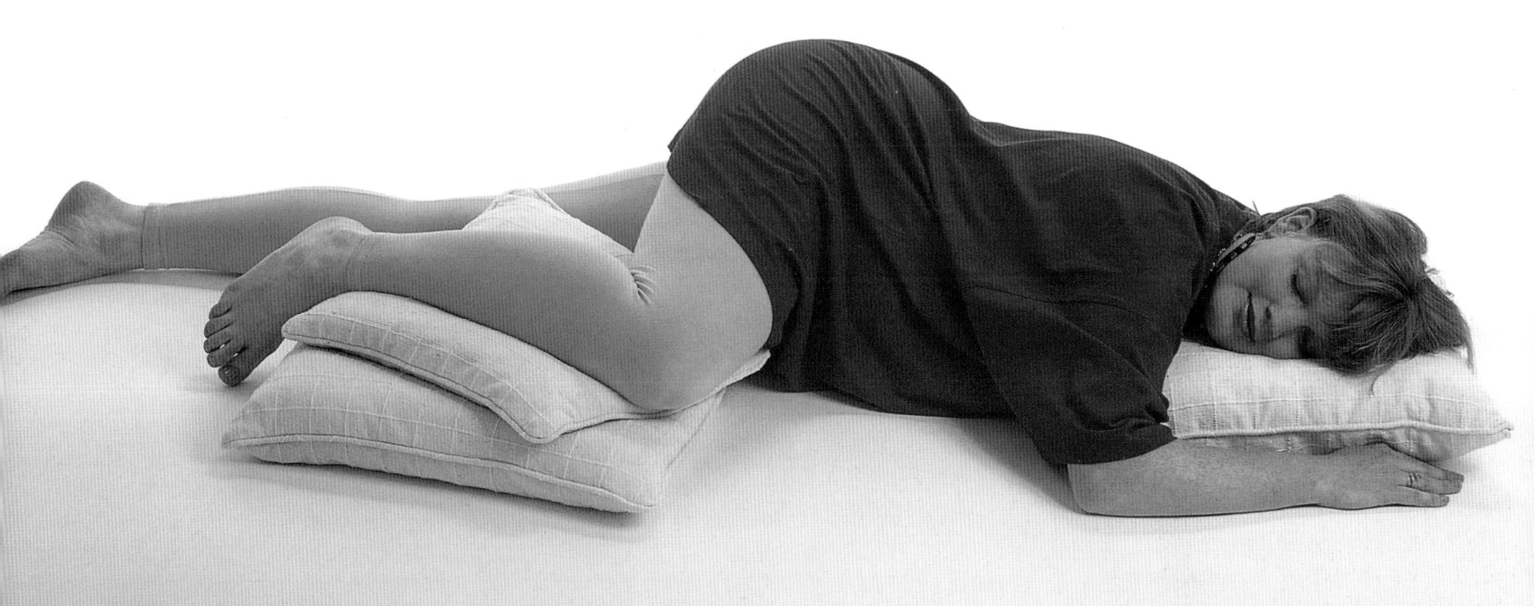

EXERCISING WITH A PARTNER

Working with another person when you exercise is fun. Not only do you involve your partner in your pregnancy, but you help each other feel relaxed and comfortable in the positions.

All of the exercises in this section are designed for two people to do together. You and your partner can even take turns between being the helper and the person exercising. You can do the exercises with another pregnant woman, with your husband or boyfriend, or with a friend or relative. They can also be introduced into a prenatal or parenting class, where several pairs work together.

What you will need

You need the same space and equipment that you've needed thus far: a simple straight-back chair, a low stool, some large cushions or a beanbag, small cushions or pillows, a bolster cushion or rolled-up blankets, plus enough empty space to work in. Wear loose, comfortable clothing. Work on a soft surface—a carpet, folded blankets, or exercise mats.

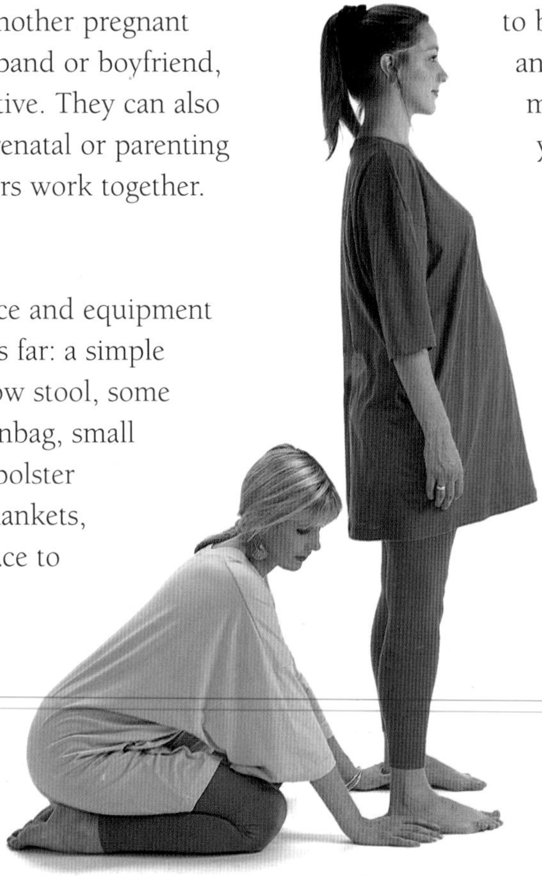

How to follow the partnership instructions

In some exercises, both partners need to follow the same instructions. In others, the instructions are different; the first set of instructions is meant for you, the pregnant woman, and the second set is for your partner. If you and another pregnant woman will be working together, it will be easier if you decide from the outset who is going to be the "partner." Stick to that formula and follow only those instructions that are meant for you. Then change roles with your partner and repeat the exercise so that you both are able to try it before moving on to the next one.

Working together

Before you start, it's a good idea to practice the communication exercise TALKING AND LISTENING (pages 68–69). This is an opportunity to let one another know how each is feeling, how your pregnancy is progressing, and what you would both like to achieve in the session. Plan the exercises that you would like to do together. Keep each other informed of one another's needs as the session progresses, and let each other know what feels really good!

Always begin your exercise session by doing some simple BREATHING (see page 12), and end with the RELAXING MASSAGE on page 93. Finish off the session with the BABY AWARENESS exercise on page 92, which can be done either relaxing in your partner's arms (as illustrated) or sitting back to back if you are working with a friend. This makes a calm, restful finish to your exercise session. Alternatively, you can practice it earlier in the session to remind you of the presence of your baby throughout.

When doing the exercises, make sure that both of you are comfortable. If the instructions involve touching or massaging your partner, be sure to work gently at first, and from time to time ask your partner how it feels.

The massages on pages 74–79, 88–91, and 93 can be done either over clothes or directly onto the skin using a light massage oil, such as almond oil. It is a good idea to warm the oil and to pour some into a bowl so that you can use it easily. All the massages are particularly relaxing if given after a warm bath, and they will help you to sleep well when done just before you go to bed.

You can also mix the partner sessions with some of the exercises that you do alone if you feel like doing a longer session, but an hour to an hour-and-a-half is long enough at any one time. A session should always end with relaxation and be followed by a drink and perhaps something to eat.

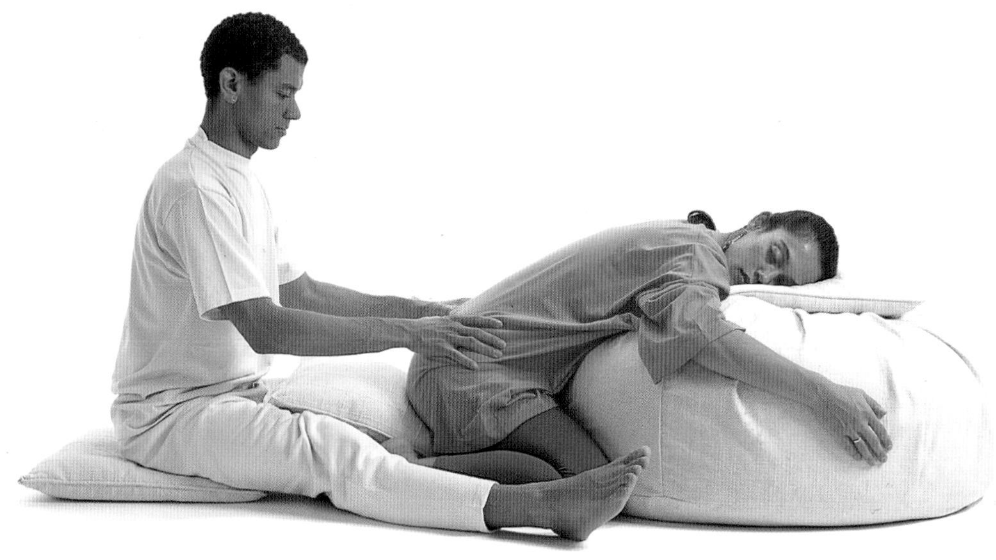

Good communication: talking and listening
Before you begin exercising together, it is always a good idea to set aside a few minutes to practice talking and listening. The exercise on the next page is an aid to open communication and will help you to develop the habit of talking about your feelings. It can be done by a couple, with a friend or relative, or in a prenatal or parenting class. After a while, it will seem less like an exercise and will come naturally, enhancing your exercise session as well as your daily life.

Start by sitting down comfortably in one of the sitting positions you have learned. Spend three to five minutes doing the breathing exercise on page 12. Then turn to face your partner—preferably close enough to touch if you are a couple.

In a group or class, divide into pairs and sit at a comfortable distance facing each other, then start by introducing yourself to your partner and telling her a little bit about yourself, your pregnancy, and your plans for the birth.

The basic principle of this exercise is that when one person talks, the other listens without interrupting. Allocate a maximum amount of time for speaking—perhaps between one and five minutes, and then take turns between listening and talking.

Begin by letting your partner know about something you appreciate and feel good about, and then go on to say how you are feeling at the moment. Then you can use the time to exchange information, to ask questions, or to let your partner know if you have any special requests or needs for the exercise session. For example you might say, "I'm very tired today and all I really want to do is to relax." Then your partner might respond, "Thanks for telling me—let's go slowly, and let me know if you want to stop or leave out any of the exercises."

This simple talking and listening technique can be used in many situations and is especially useful when conflict arises or if there are any disagreements in a relationship. If you can develop the habit of talking and listening to each other in a calm and balanced way, you will find that most problems can be solved and that you can cope with anything that may happen. It is also a great way to share your wishes, hopes, and dreams.

In a group, it is an enjoyable way to get to others better and to make new friends. You can also use this exercise at home within your family, and later on, it will help you to communicate successfully with your child.

TALKING AND LISTENING

This communication exercise will help you develop the habit of sharing your feelings.

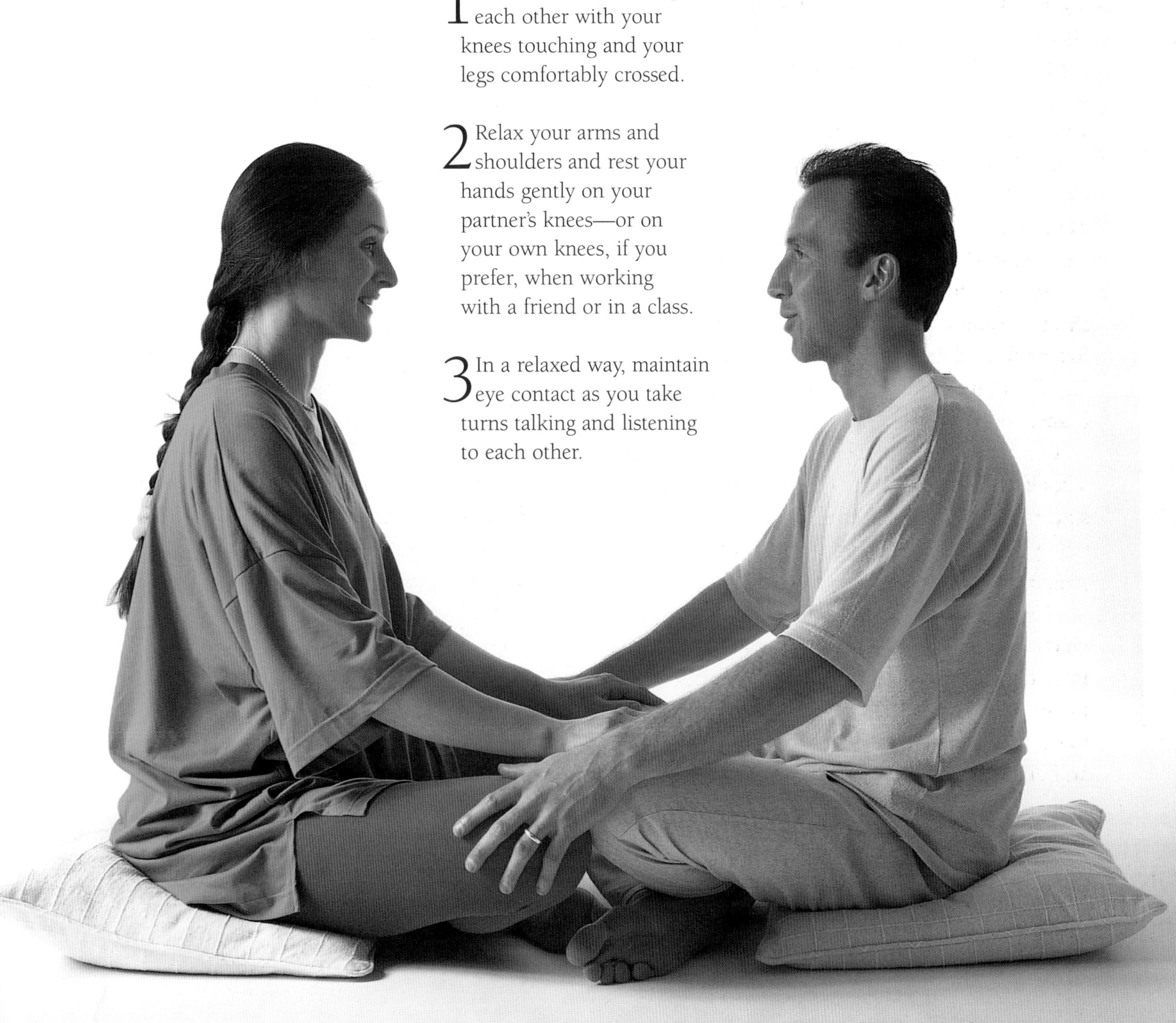

1 Sit on a cushion facing each other with your knees touching and your legs comfortably crossed.

2 Relax your arms and shoulders and rest your hands gently on your partner's knees—or on your own knees, if you prefer, when working with a friend or in a class.

3 In a relaxed way, maintain eye contact as you take turns talking and listening to each other.

LEG SPREAD—BACK TO BACK

Working together back to back gives you support in the lower back, allowing the weight of your pelvis and legs to relax onto the floor while your shoulders and spine feel light and free.

1 Sit back to back with your lower backs touching, and spread your legs as wide apart as you comfortably can.

2 Allow your upper back, between the shoulder blades, to make light contact with that of your partner.

3 Relax your shoulders, and place your hands gently on your thighs.

4 Focus on your breathing. Feel the weight of your pelvis and legs slowly sink toward the ground each time you exhale. Allow your spine to lengthen gently toward the ceiling as you breathe in.

5 Remain in this position for up to three minutes or until one of you wants to stop.

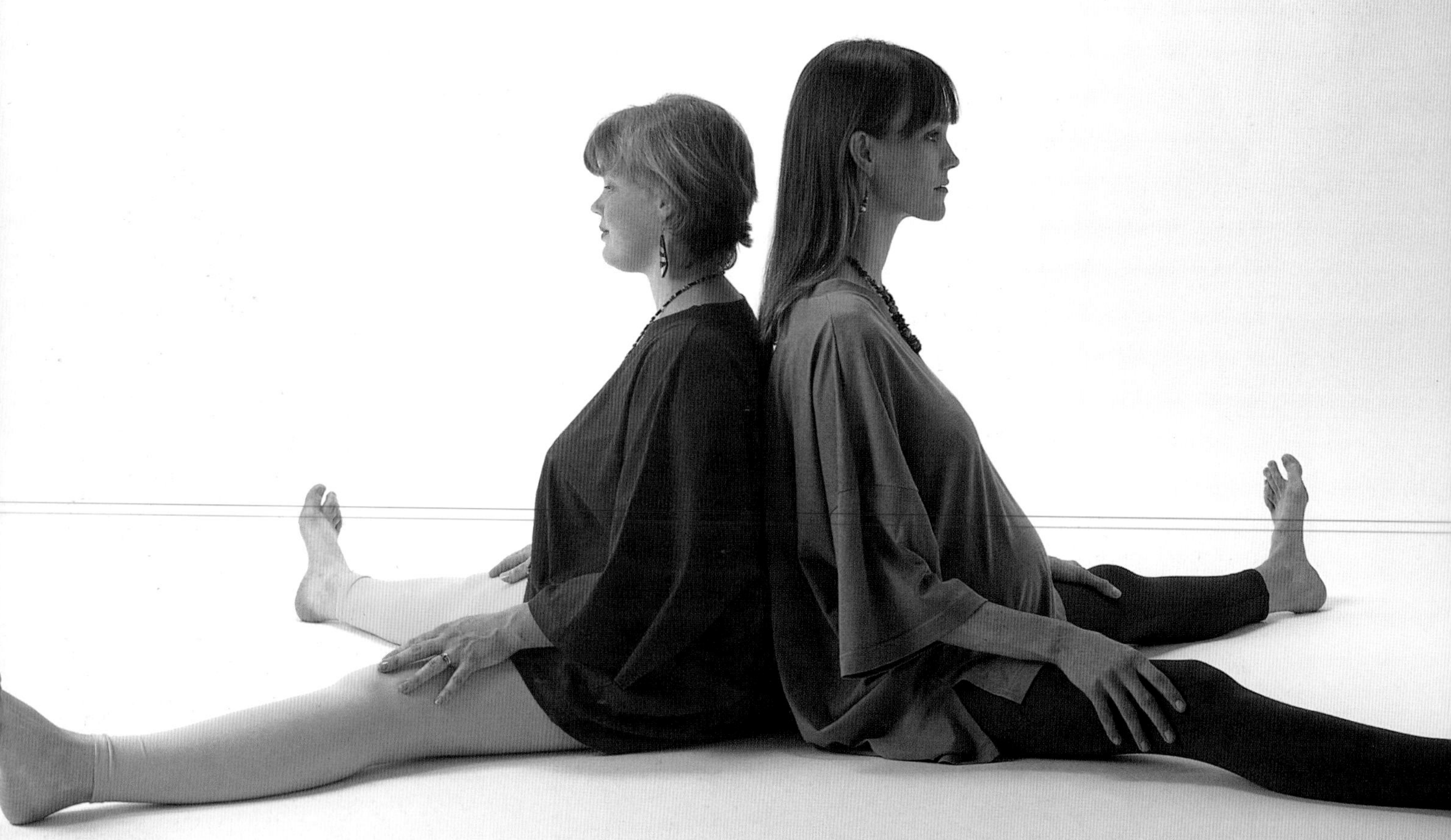

LEG SPREAD—FEET IN THE BACK

Some people find this more comfortable than the exercise on the opposite page, and it supports your lower back in a similar way.

1 Sit with your legs spread wide apart and let your partner's feet support your lower back.

2 Relax in the position for a minute or so, releasing the back of your neck by tilting your head slightly forward.

3 Continue to focus on the natural flow of your breathing.

4 To come out of the position, slowly bring your legs together with the help of your hands, and then move away from your partner.

Partner

1 Place the soles of your feet firmly against your partner's lower back.

2 Straighten your legs and lean back slightly, supporting yourself with your hands. Keep your shoulders relaxed and make sure that you feel comfortable.

3 Breathing evenly, gently increase the pressure of your feet until your partner feels well supported.

4 Focus on your breathing and the downward pull of gravity through your legs.

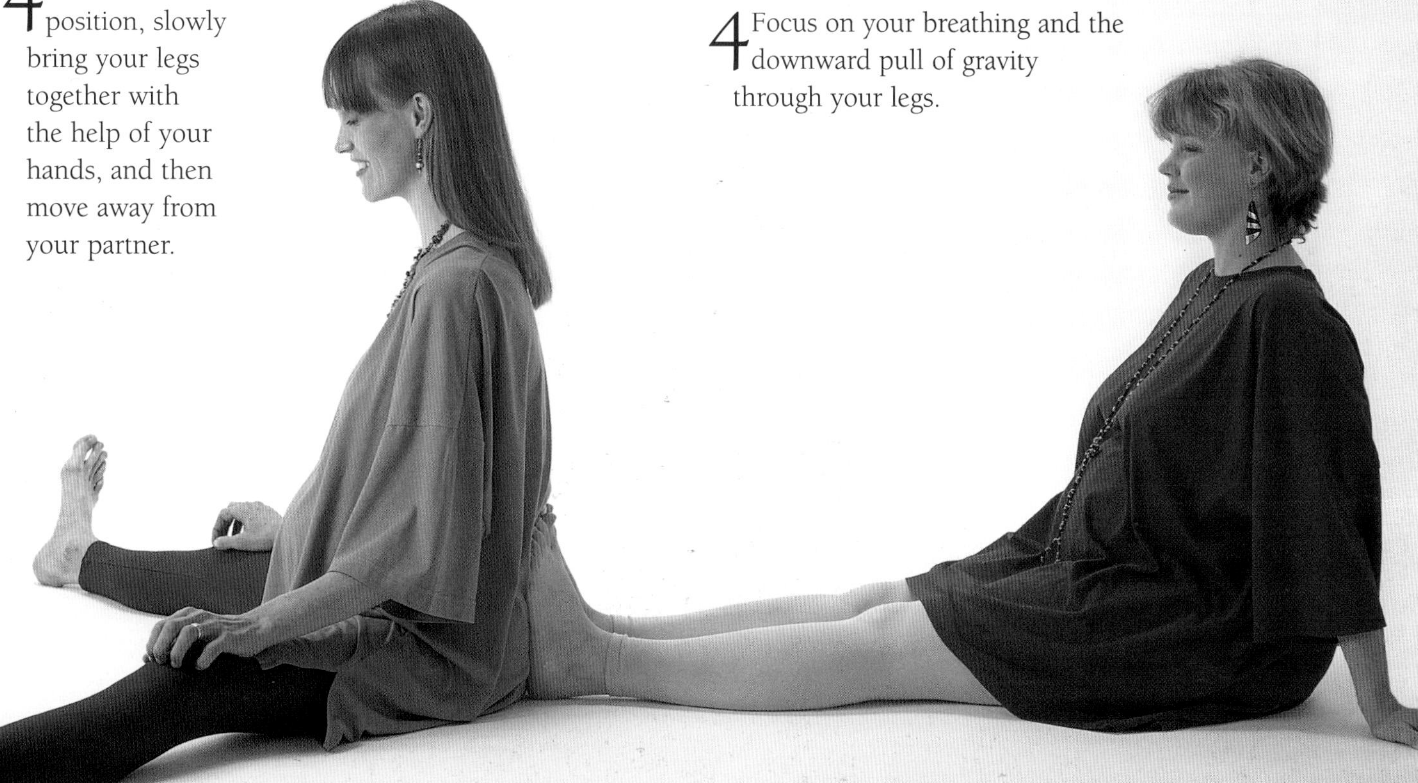

TAILOR POSITION—BACK TO BACK

This is a warm, friendly way to practice tailor sitting with your back supported comfortably.

1 Bring your lower back as close to your partner's as possible.

2 Bend your knees, and place the soles of your feet together at a comfortable distance from your body.

3 Place a cushion or two under your knees so that your legs are well supported and you can relax.

4 Relax your shoulders and feel your upper back making gentle contact with your partner. Relax your arms and place your hands on your calves.

5 Close your eyes and focus on your breathing. Feel your lower back and hips release toward the floor while your spine lengthens from the back of your waist to the top of your neck.

Remember

Avoid leaning heavily against your partner, bouncing your knees, or pulling your legs in too close to your body.

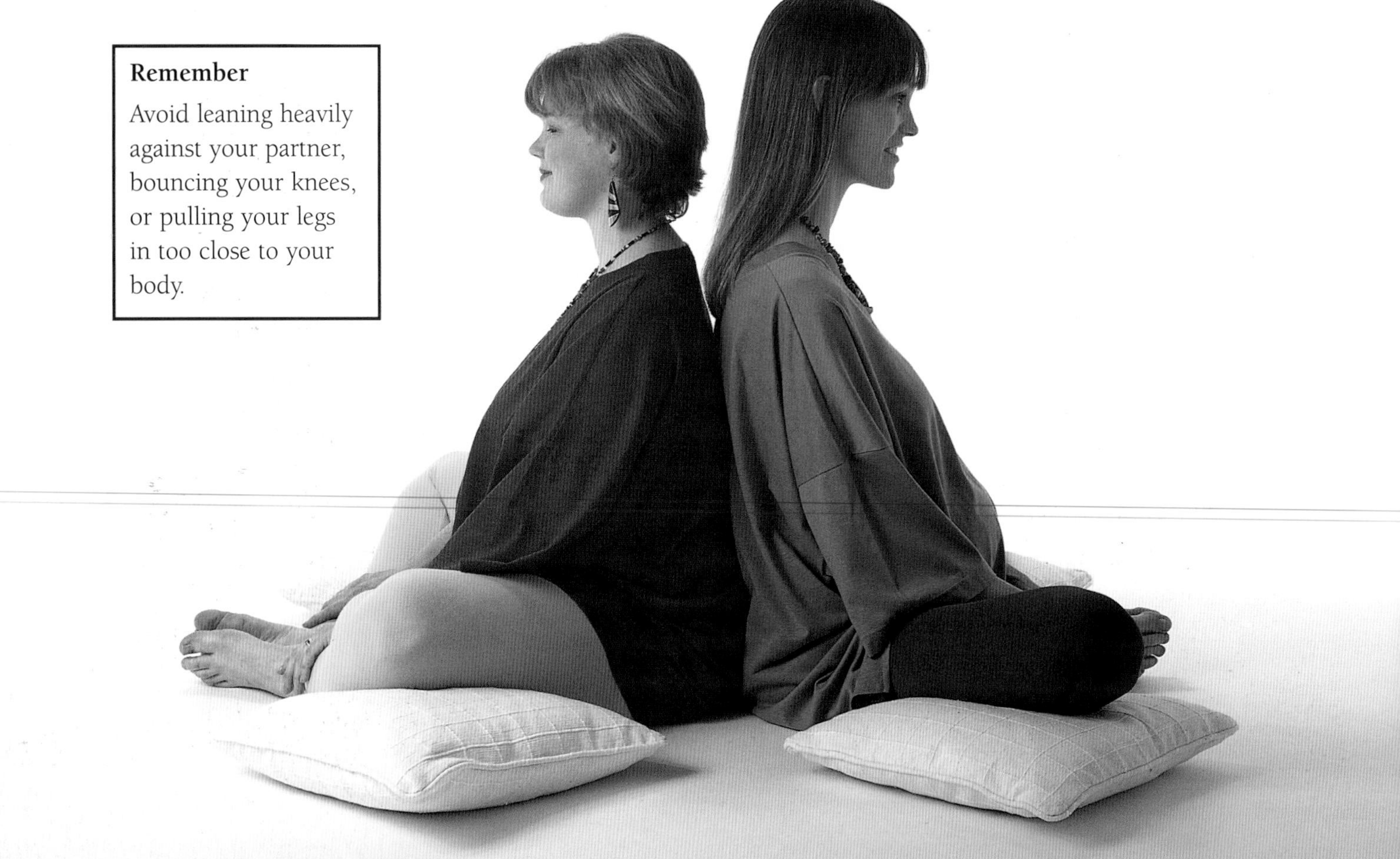

TAILOR POSITION—FEET IN THE BACK

This is a very comfortable way to be supported while tailor sitting.

1 Bend your knees, and place the soles of your feet together at a comfortable distance from your body.

2 Use cushions to support your legs, unless they rest comfortably on the ground.

3 Relax and focus on your breathing rhythm for a minute or two.

Partner

1 Place the soles of your feet firmly against the lower back of your partner.

2 Straighten your legs and lean back slightly, supporting yourself with your hands.

3 Gently increase the pressure from your feet until your partner is well supported.

4 Focus on your breathing and on the downward pull of gravity through your legs.

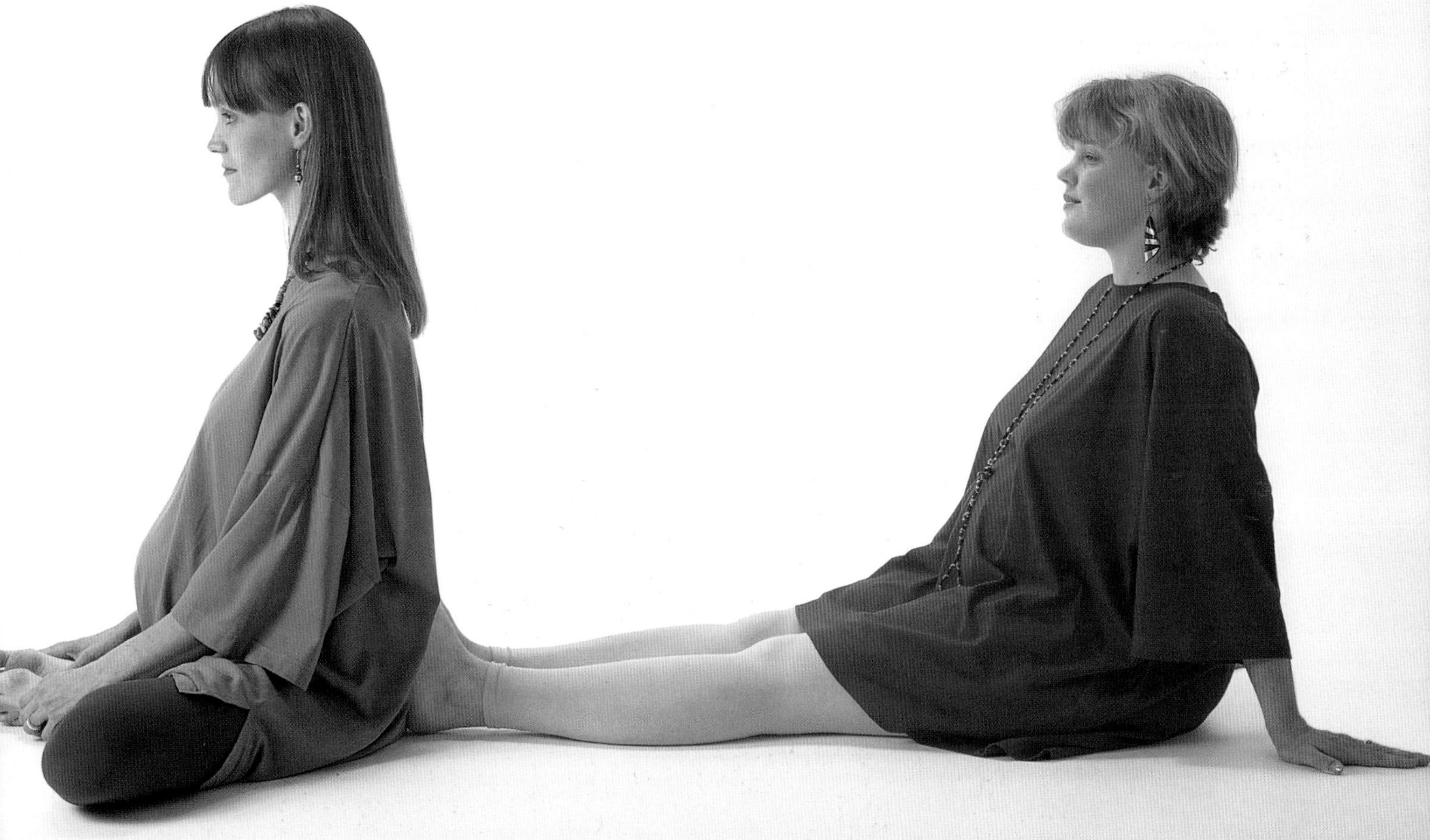

KNEELING

SHOULDER MASSAGE

The exercises on pages 74–79 can be done separately or as one massage sequence. Practice all of them on a soft surface suitable for kneeling, and use a long cushion or bolster, plus several small cushions if necessary, so that your hips are raised slightly higher than your knees and are well supported throughout. Place a beanbag and a cushion in front of you in preparation for the later exercises.

1 Kneel in the UPRIGHT CHILD'S POSE (page 32) and relax. Close your eyes and focus on your breathing.

2 Release your lower back downward, following the curve of the bones at the base of your spine. Feel your weight settle in your pelvis.

3 Gently lengthen your spine toward the top of your neck, and slightly release your chin downward. Relax your jaw and your shoulders as your partner begins the massage.

Partner

1 Place a cushion on a low stool, and sit comfortably behind your partner. Gently place your hands on her shoulders.

2 Focus on your breathing, and notice how her muscles feel under your hands.

3 Massage her shoulders with a relaxed kneading movement, applying the amount of pressure that feels comfortable to her.

4 Continue for a minute or two, working gently from the top of the neck, then to the upper back, shoulder blades, and arms.

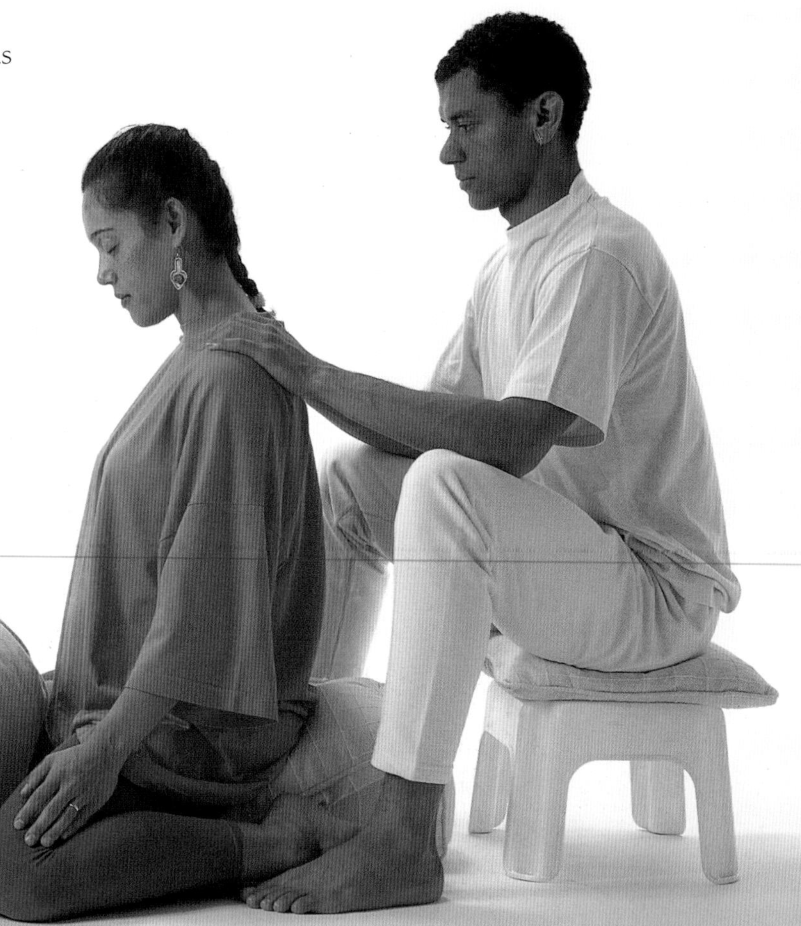

LOWER BACK RELEASE

This movement keeps the pelvis well grounded, allowing the spine to lengthen as the shoulders release and the arms come up.

1 Be aware of your breathing and release your lower back downward.

2 As your partner holds your hips, slowly raise both arms up over your head, keeping your elbows slightly bent and your shoulders down.

3 Hold the position for a few moments, and then slowly lower your arms.

Partner

1 Sit behind your partner, on a small cushion on the floor. Your legs should be spread apart so that you feel comfortable and relaxed.

2 Place your hands around your partner's pelvic bones so that they rest securely on the rim.

3 Gently exert a continuous downward pressure to encourage the pelvis to relax.

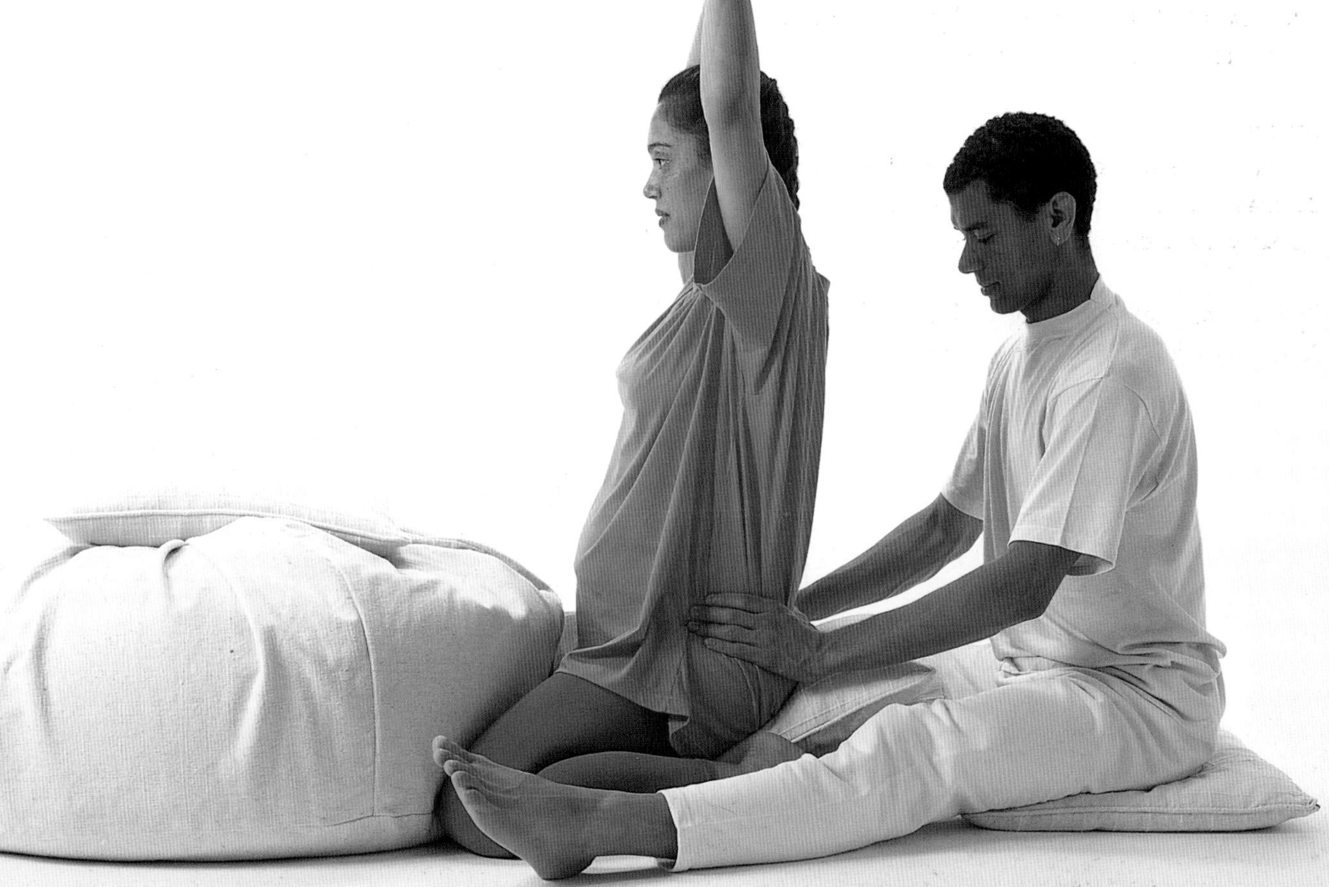

LOWER BACK MASSAGE

Leaning forward onto a beanbag takes the weight off your lower back and is a perfect position for a massage. While you are relaxing, this position is also helping to guide your baby into a good position for birth and is releasing tension in the groin, hips, knees, and ankles.

1 Slowly lean forward from your hips, and relax onto the beanbag with your upper body comfortably supported.

2 Turn your head to one side and rest it on the beanbag, with your neck relaxed and your eyes closed. Relax your shoulders, and spread your arms out to the sides.

3 Focus on your breathing and relax completely, allowing yourself to sink into a peaceful state as your partner works.

Partner

1 Gently hold your partner's pelvis down as she moves forward.

2 Place both of your hands over her lower back, and pause for a moment or two, focusing on your breathing and the sensations in your hands.

3 Once your partner is relaxed and comfortable, begin to work with your thumbs, massaging over the pelvic bones.

4 Use both of your hands to circle up the center of her lower back and then around her sides, hips, and buttocks.

5 Continue doing this for a minute or two, making smooth, soothing movements.

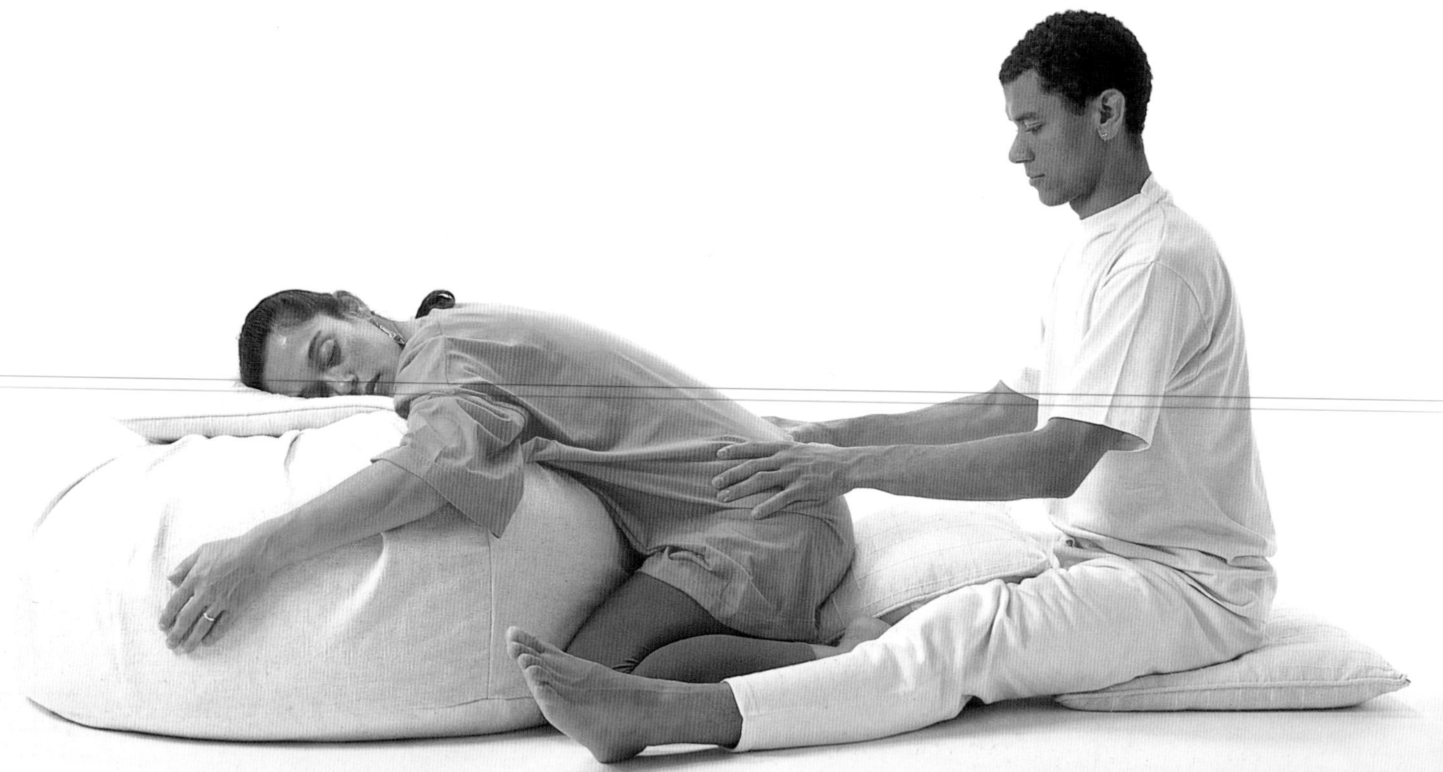

LONG STROKES

These strokes relax the long muscles that run down either side of the spine, and move the energy from the head and shoulders down toward the pelvis. This helps to release tension in the upper body.

1 Rest on the beanbag as shown on the opposite page and continue breathing and relaxing while your partner works.

Partner

1 Kneel with one knee on a cushion and the other one raised, so that you are comfortable.

2 Using one hand and then the other in a smooth alternating rhythm, stroke down your partner's spine from her neck to her tailbone.

3 Continue in this way for a minute or so, stroking slowly and gently, and end by resting both hands on your partner's lower back.

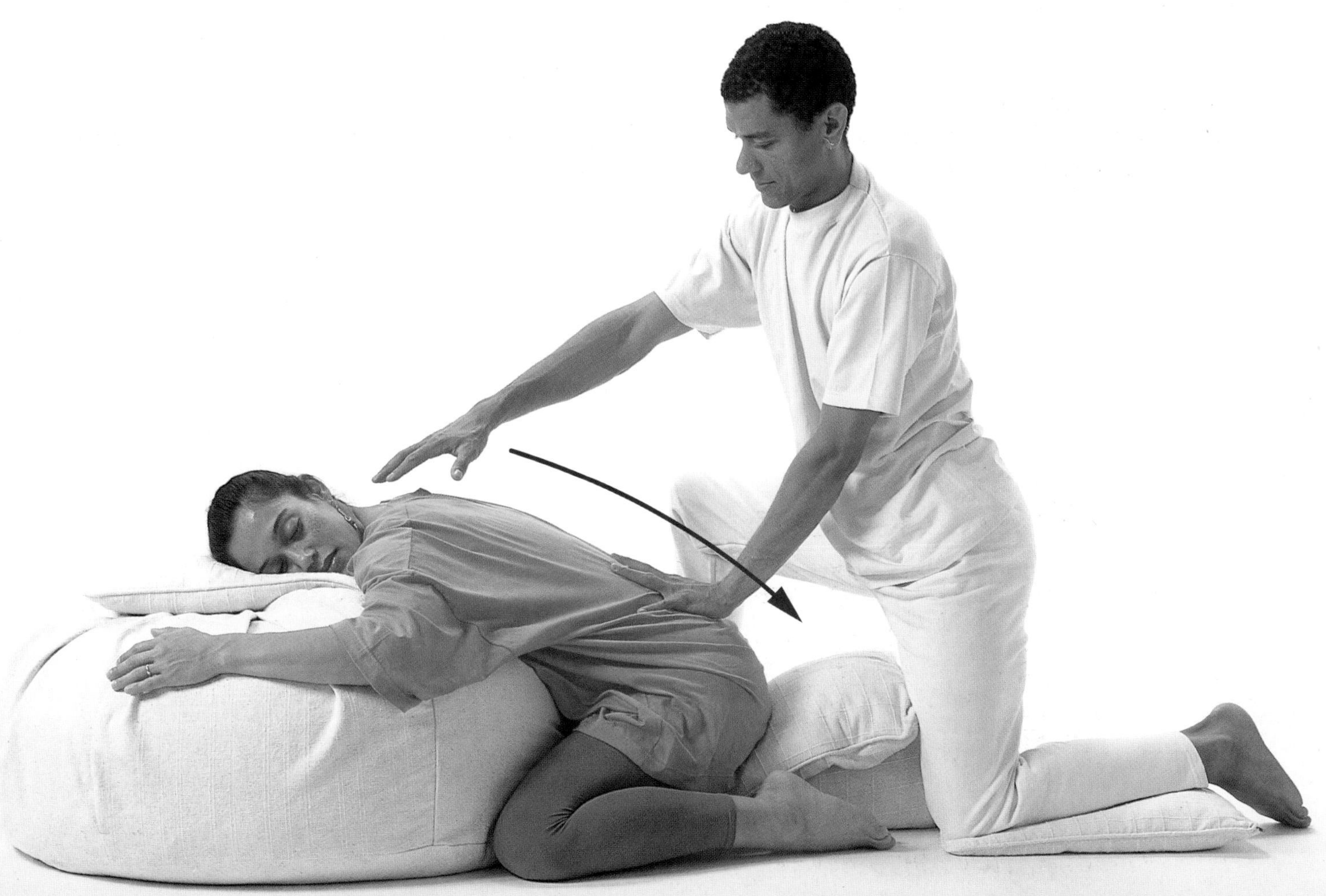

FULL BODY STROKES

This wonderful massage stroke was invented by a father whom I taught many years ago. He used it throughout labor to alleviate the pain. In pregnancy, it is very comforting and relaxing, releasing tension and fatigue throughout the entire body.

1 Rest on a beanbag as shown on page 76. Breathe and relax while your partner works.

Partner

1 Kneel as shown in the exercise on page 77, and place your left hand on your partner's left shoulder. Your palm should be flat and your fingers should be relaxed.

2 As your partner exhales, slowly stroke down the left side of her spine. In one continuous movement, go around her left hip, along her thigh, around her knee, along her calf, and out through her toes.

3 Flick your hand to discharge the energy, and repeat the same movement with your right hand on your partner's right side.

4 Continue alternating the left and right sides until you have done three strokes on each side. Repeat the movement three times with both of your hands down both of your partner's sides simultaneously.

5 Repeat this whole sequence two or three times, and end by resting both of your hands on her lower back.

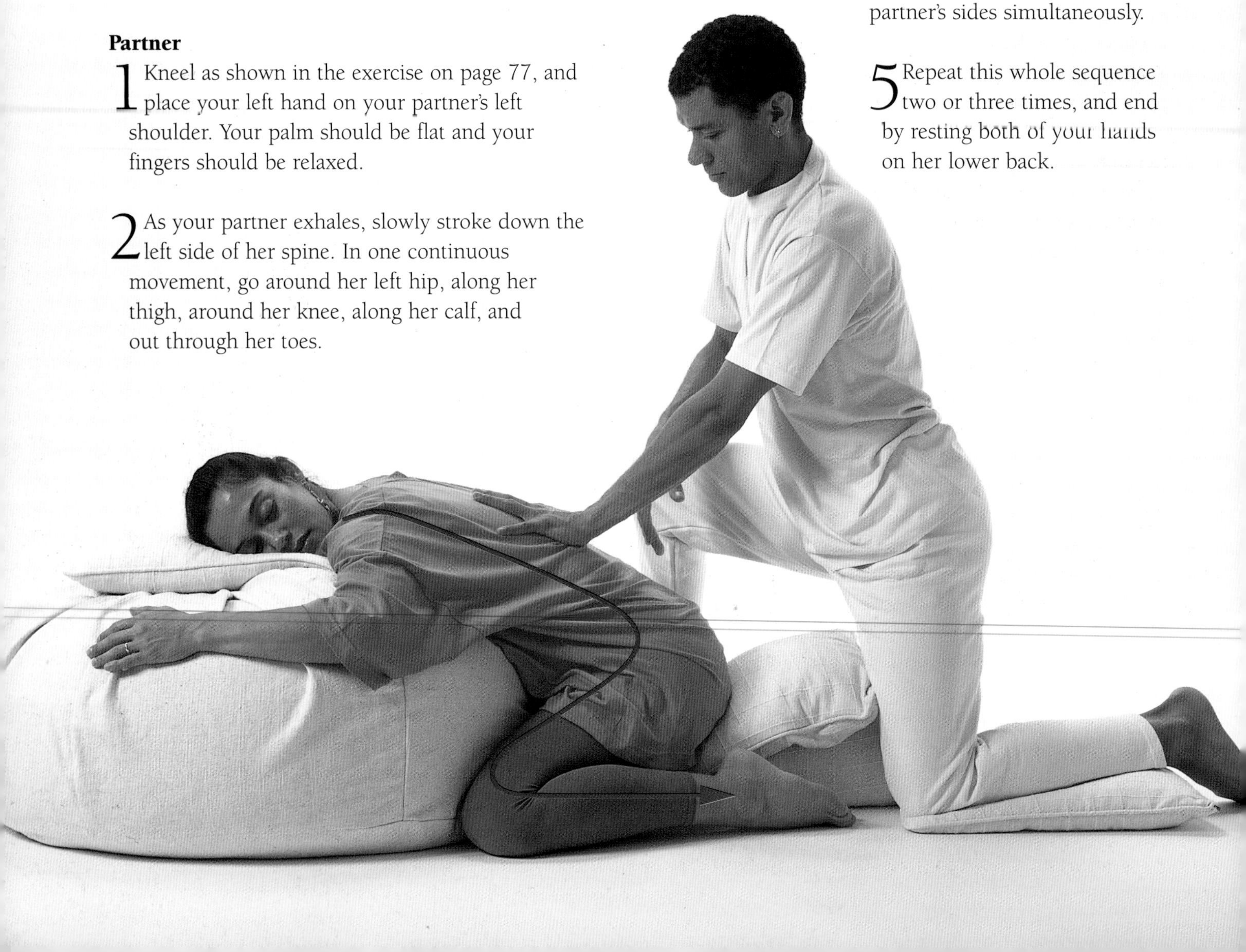

COMING UP SLOWLY

Slowly returning to the vertical position as you do in this exercise allows the weight to settle in your pelvis and the heavy base of your spine before the rest of your spine gradually lengthens upward toward the neck. This creates a feeling of relaxation and release in the neck and shoulders and a sense of lightness in the upper body.

1 Focusing on your pelvis, breathe evenly as you begin to release the curve of your lower back downward with the help of your partner.

2 Curl up to the vertical position, starting from the base and slowly working upward so that your shoulders, neck, and head come up last.

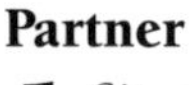

Partner

1 Sit or kneel comfortably behind your partner, and place both hands firmly over the base of her spine.

2 To encourage the lower back to drop first, exert a gentle downward pressure as your partner begins to rise, and then stroke down her spine as it lengthens.

3 Once her spine is vertical, remove your hands. End with a brief massage of her shoulders and arms.

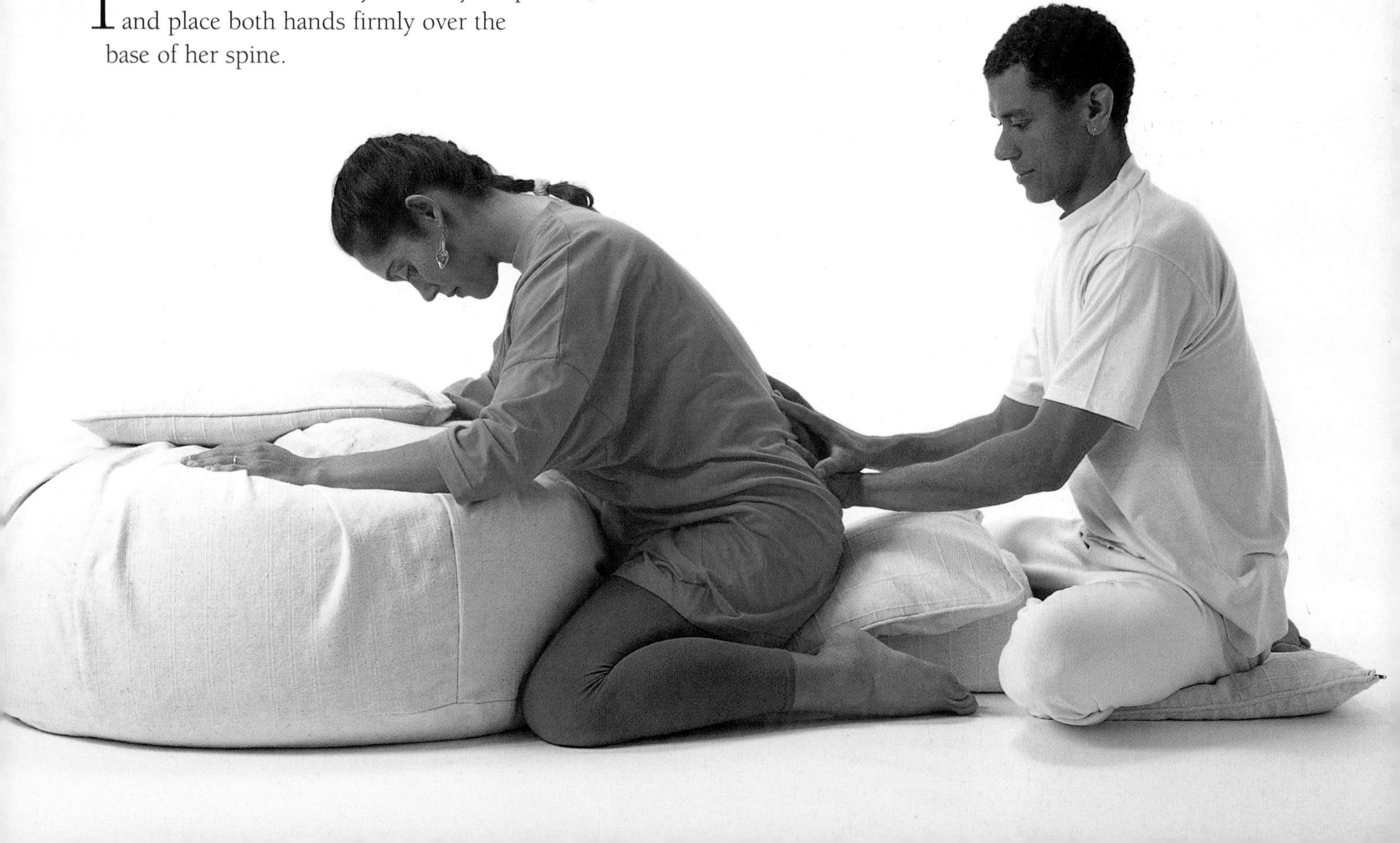

GROUNDING

Working with a partner while doing this exercise helps your body to feel well grounded from the feet up to the waist, while the upper body responds by relaxing as tension releases from your neck and shoulders. The pull of gravity anchoring you to the ground helps you to be aware of your standing and walking posture.

1 Stand with your feet about twelve inches (hips' width) apart, with your heels slightly wider apart than your toes.

2 Focus on your breathing, and relax the soles of your feet, sensing the ground underneath you.

3 Feel your weight fall evenly through both heels, and release your lower back downward.

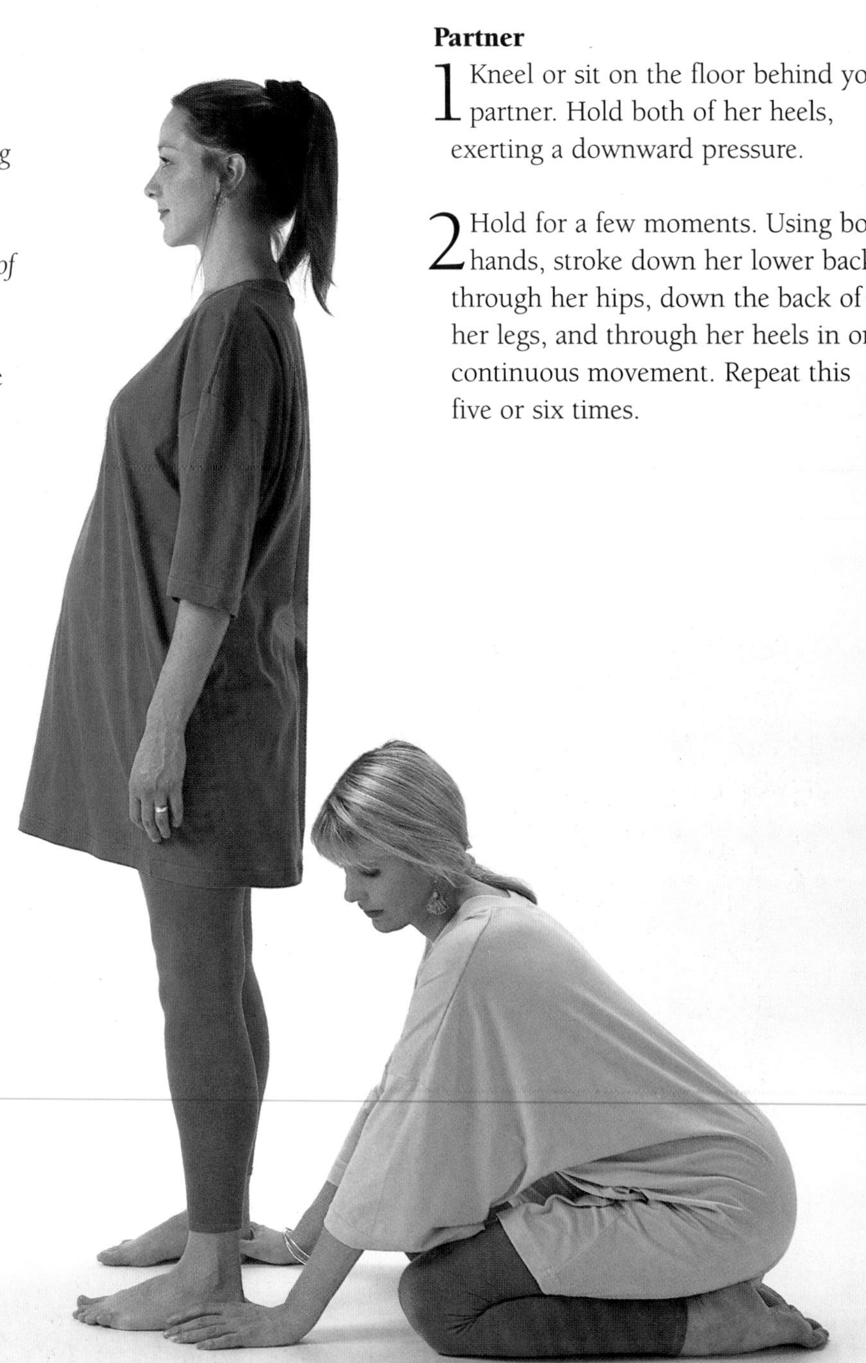

Partner

1 Kneel or sit on the floor behind your partner. Hold both of her heels, exerting a downward pressure.

2 Hold for a few moments. Using both hands, stroke down her lower back, through her hips, down the back of her legs, and through her heels in one continuous movement. Repeat this five or six times.

BENDING FORWARD

This forward bend releases tension in the hamstring muscles at the back of the legs, lengthens the spine, and relaxes the shoulders.

Remember

Omit this exercise if you feel uncomfortable or light-headed when you bend forward or if you have painful hemorrhoids.

1 Stand as in the GROUNDING exercise on the opposite page, facing your partner. Press your weight through your heels, and lean forward slowly from your hips until your torso is parallel to the floor.

2 Extend both arms, keeping your elbows straight. As your partner supports you, relax your shoulders and gently lengthen your spine. Keep releasing your weight through your heels, and breathe evenly.

3 Hold for a few moments, and slowly return to the vertical position. Plant your heels, bend your knees, and curl up slowly, first releasing your lower back downward and coming up from the base of the spine.

Partner

1 Face your partner with your feet parallel and your lower back releasing downward.

2 When your partner bends forward, gently support her wrists from underneath without bending your own back or leaning forward.

CALF STRETCH

This exercise lengthens the calf muscles and the back of the heels, helping to increase flexibility in the ankles. This makes squatting easier and can also relieve cramps in the calves.

1 Stand facing a wall in the GOOD STANDING or GROUNDING positions (pages 40 or 80) at an arm's distance from the wall.

2 Place your right leg forward and left leg back, bending your right knee and keeping your left knee straight Your heels should be down on the ground. Both feet remain parallel.

3 Keeping your hips parallel to the wall, clasp your hands and lean forward onto your forearms and elbows, with your neck and shoulders relaxed. Breathe evenly, feeling the stretch in the back of your left leg.

4 Hold for three cycles of the breathing rhythm and then switch sides. Repeat on both legs twice.

Partner

1 Kneel or sit comfortably behind your partner.

2 Use your left hand to hold your partner's heel, pressing down gently but firmly. Your right hand should support the front of her knee, gently encouraging the back of her leg to open.

3 Hold until your partner switches legs, and then repeat on the other side reversing your hand positions.

SUPPORTING FROM BEHIND

Regularly practicing your squatting will help you to be at ease in supported squat positions during labour and birth by slowly increasing the flexibility of your hips, knees, and ankles and by strengthening your thighs.

1 Place your feet a little wider apart than in your normal standing position, and slightly turned out. Position a bolster, a pile of books, or a low stool between your legs. Breathe evenly.

2 With your partner behind you, bend your knees, and, keeping both heels down on the floor, slowly lower your pelvis into the squatting position.

3 Hold for a minute or two, and then rise by pressing your heels down, slowly raising your pelvis, and straightening your legs. Alternatively, you can come forward onto your hands and knees before coming up. Repeat once or twice.

Partner

1 Stand behind your partner so that her lower back is supported by your legs. Breathe evenly.

2 Bend forward from your hips, keeping your own back relaxed, and place your hands on your partner's knees. Relax your neck and shoulders, and lean softly down onto her knees to create a gentle sense of downward pressure toward her heels.

3 To assist your partner as she rises, support her rib cage on both sides with your hands gently, just under her arms.

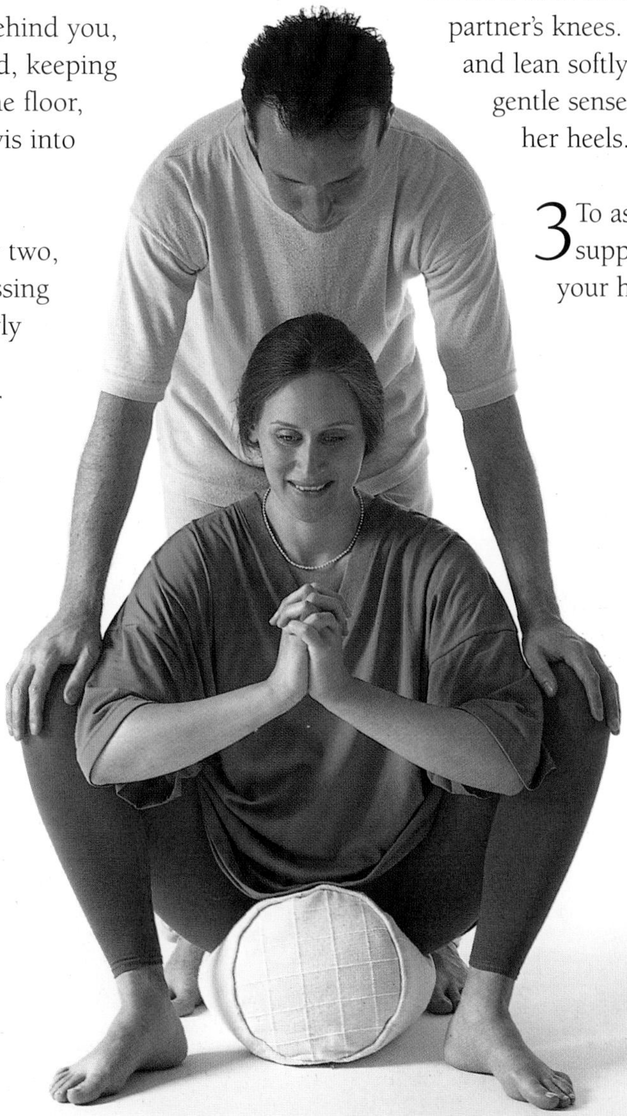

Remember

Avoid deep squats in the last six weeks of pregnancy. Omit the partner squats on pages 83–85 until your doctor or midwife has confirmed that your baby's head has fully engaged.

If you have weak or painful knees, use a low stool under your pelvis, and avoid deep squats.

PARTNER ON A CHAIR

This is an easy way to practice squatting and also can be used occasionally during labor to strengthen contractions or as a birthing position.

1 Stand facing your partner as is shown on page 83. Hold each other by the wrists so that both of you have your arms outstretched.

2 Keep your heels on the floor, bend your knees, and slowly lower your pelvis until your buttocks rest on the support. Make sure that you are far enough from your partner so that both of you can keep your arms straight.

3 Relax and lengthen your back and neck, and hold for three to five cycles of the breathing rhythm. Slowly stand up by planting your heels down, and gradually raising your pelvis and straightening your legs. Repeat this twice.

Partner

1 Hold your partner by the wrists. Sit securely on a chair, with your feet well grounded and your knees comfortably apart. Relax your lower back toward the seat of the chair, and breathe evenly.

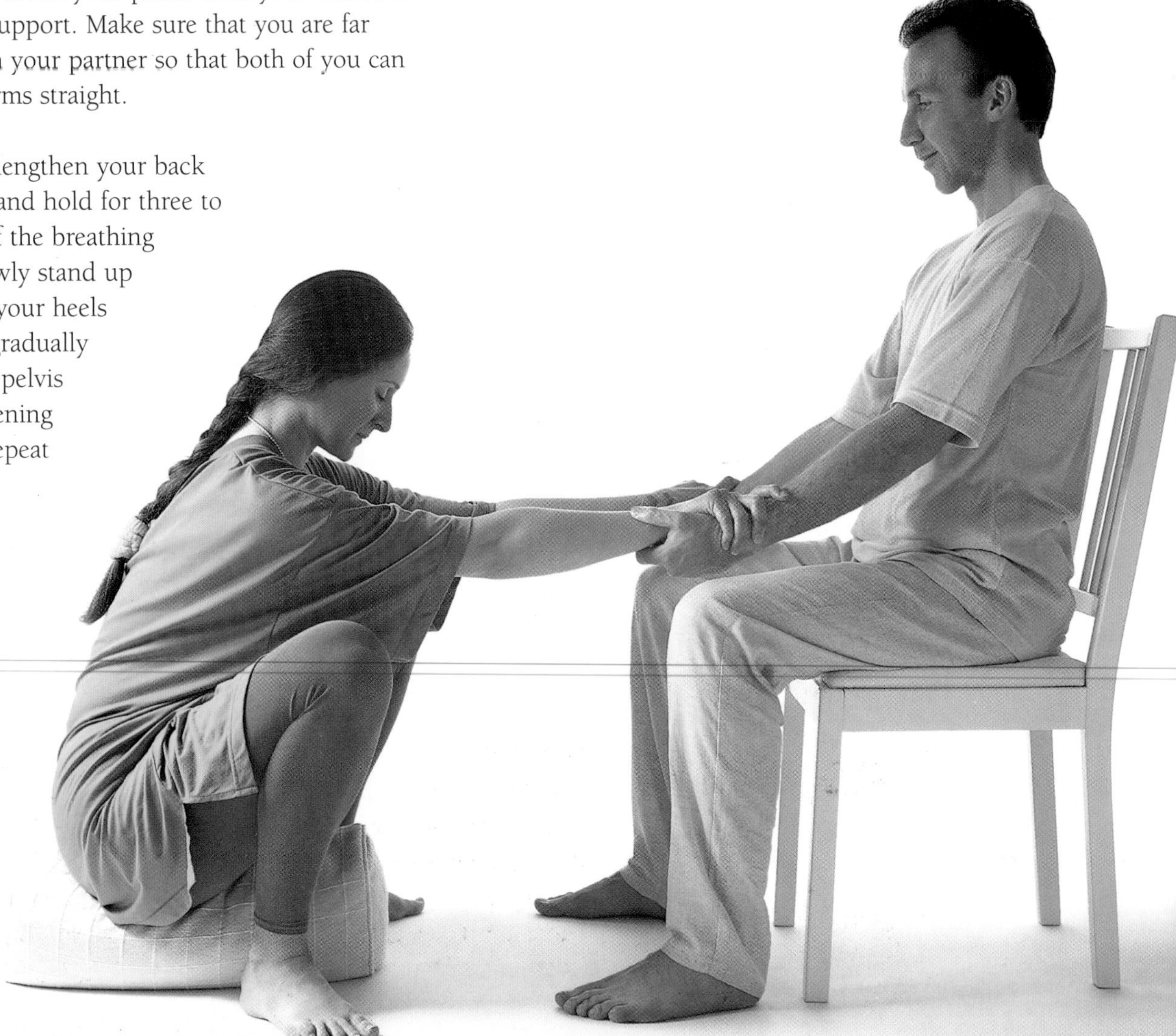

SQUATTING TOGETHER

This way of practicing squatting is more challenging, so omit it if you find squatting to be difficult. You can also make it easier if both or one of you uses the support of a bolster or stool.

1 Stand facing each other, and hold each other firmly by the wrists with your arms outstretched and your elbows straight. Place your feet slightly wider apart than your usual standing position, and slightly turn them out.

2 Keeping your heels down, and breathing evenly, slowly bend your knees and lower your pelvis into a squat. Make sure that you are far enough away from your partner to pull gently on each other for support with your back relaxed, heels down, and arms straight.

3 Hold for a short time and then slowly rise together, still holding on to each other. As you come up, press your heels down into the ground, gently raise your pelvis, and slowly straighten your legs. Rest and repeat twice.

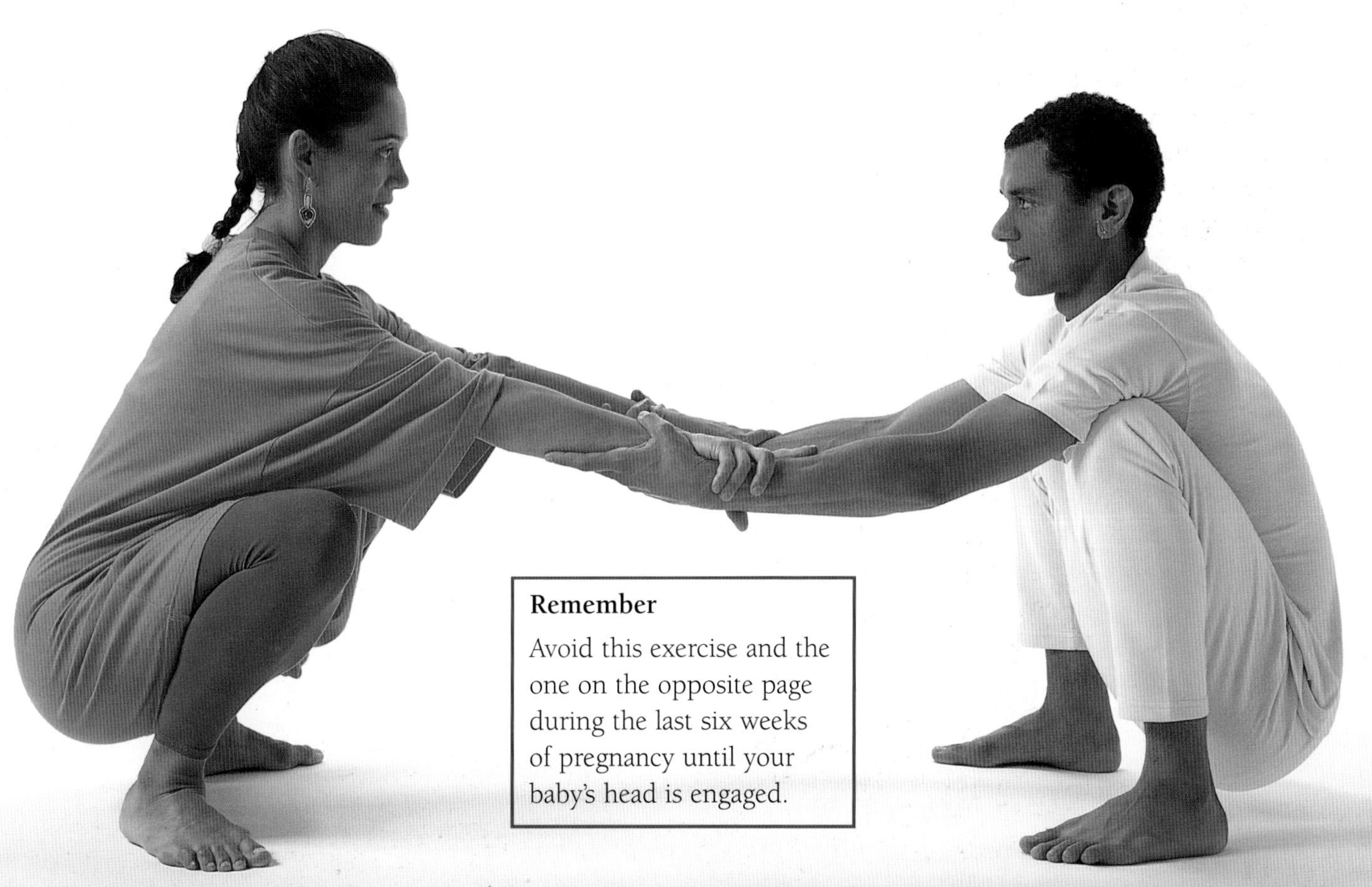

Remember

Avoid this exercise and the one on the opposite page during the last six weeks of pregnancy until your baby's head is engaged.

MASSAGE FOR LABOR

If you are planning to share your labor with a partner, it's a good idea to do some practicing together throughout your pregnancy, especially in the last six weeks. The following exercises involve massage and can be practiced over your clothes. Sometimes, however, it is helpful and enjoyable to work directly on the skin using a mild massage oil. This will prepare you for working in labor, when the skin may become irritated by massage over clothing; in this case, it is better to work with oil on the skin.

Preparing for massage

Create an atmosphere in which you both feel comfortable, with low lighting or candlelight and perhaps some soothing music in the background, at a time when you won't be interrupted. Make sure the room is warm—though not too warm—and pleasant to be in. You can do this session at any time, but it's especially enjoyable after a bath just before going to bed.

Start by spending ten minutes together doing the BREATHING and BABY AWARENESS exercises (see pages 12, 13, and 91). Tune in to the presence of your baby so that you are conscious of your child being there with you throughout. It is as important to be able to be silent and peaceful together, without doing anything else, as it is to do practical things, so take your time before you start.

Massage in pregnancy

The exercises that follow suggest some simple massage techniques that can be used in labor. Many women find that massage in labor is helpful for comfort and pain relief, while others prefer not to be touched. It is impossible to predict whether this sort of help will be useful at the time. However, since most women find massage enjoyable in late pregnancy, it is worth doing now, even if during labor you decide you don't want to be massaged. Massage will help you to develop the art of communicating through touch and will enhance your relationship. Once you get used to being massaged in kneeling or standing positions, try alternatives such as sitting backward on a chair, resting your upper body, arms and head on a pillow, or kneeling over a beanbag.

The massaging partner

If you are the partner giving the massage, it is important for you to also be comfortable. Wear light, loose-fitting clothing, and, if it helps you feel more relaxed, use a low stool, some cushions, or a bolster to sit on as you work.

Make sure your arms and shoulders are relaxed, your back feels loose and comfortable, and your hands are warm. Take your time before starting to massage your partner. First focus on your own breathing and notice how your body feels. Then pause to release any tension that you have become aware of in your neck, shoulders, arms, or legs.

When you are ready, very slowly bring your hands into contact with your partner's body, and gently start the massage. After a while, ask her how it feels, whether she would like more or less pressure, and whether your hands are in the right place. You will find, in time, that these sessions are so enjoyable that you will soon become a confident and intuitive masseur, developing your own style and method of helping your partner with a touch that is sensitive to her needs.

Keep the massage simple and relaxed, concentrating on soothing movements that help to take away pain. You will notice that the massage strokes shown here focus on the lower back. This is because the sacral nerves from the uterus go up through the lower back into the spinal cord toward the brain. When you massage this area during a contraction in labor, the pleasant sensations you are creating travel to the brain and help to positively influence your partner's perception of the pain. However, if you notice that her shoulders look tense, then use your intuition and work for a while on her shoulders, or try the FULL BODY STROKES technique shown on page 78, using oil on the skin. It is usually best to massage during the contractions, and to rest in between them.

Sharing your feelings

When you practice, change positions from time to time so that your partner receives a massage, too. This is a creative way to exchange ideas and information about ways you like to be touched. You should complete your massage session with the TALKING AND LISTENING exercise on page 69. Start by telling each other all the things you appreciated about the massage. Then take turns sharing information about anything you would like to change the next time. Recommend specifically how you would like your partner to work—ideally with a demonstration. End by thanking each other and planning a time for your next practice session. You may also want to do the relaxation exercises on pages 92 and 93.

CIRCLING

1 On a soft surface, kneel in the all-fours position or over a beanbag. Make sure your neck and shoulders are relaxed and that there is no discomfort in your wrists.

2 Inhale through your nose and slowly exhale through your mouth, as if you were in labor, while moving your body or circling your hips rhythmically as your partner is working.

3 Continue doing this for a minute or two and rise slowly when you are ready. Rest and then repeat once or twice.

Partner

1 Kneel behind your partner or sit on a stool for support. Place both hands gently on her lower back and breathe evenly, relaxing your hands.

2 Slowly make a circular movement with both of your hands, stroking up her lower back toward her waistline, and then around her hips and back to the center. Continue like this for a minute or two with a smooth, even pressure.

3 Using only one hand, make a broader circle around your partner's lower back and hips. Continue until she is ready to rise.

4 Repeat both of these massage strokes one more time, but first ask how it felt.

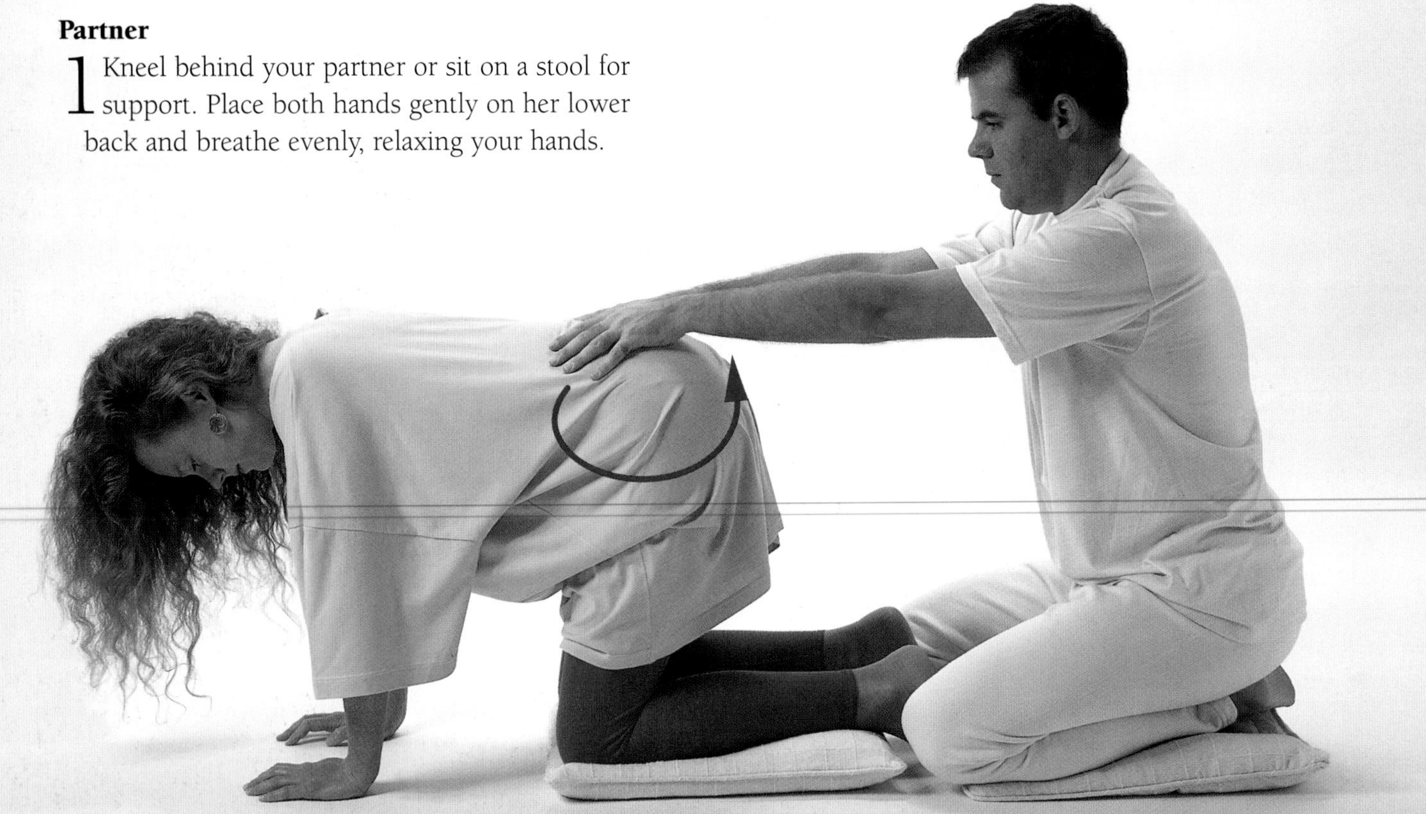

BASE OF THE SPINE

1 On a soft surface, kneel either in the all-fours position or over a beanbag. Make sure your neck and shoulders are relaxed and that there is no discomfort in your wrists.

2 Lean backward toward your partner's hand, using the pressure to create a gentle sense of resistance. This may help to relieve pain during contractions in labor.

3 Continue doing this for a minute or so and then rise.

Partner

1 Kneel behind your partner with one leg raised, and place the palm of one hand over her lower back so that her tailbone rests just below the heel of your palm.

2 Keep your elbow straight, and gently lean your body weight toward your hand, providing an even pressure for your partner to lean into.

3 Allow your partner to move and do the work while you simply offer gentle resistance.

4 Keep your hand in this position for a minute or two and then rest.

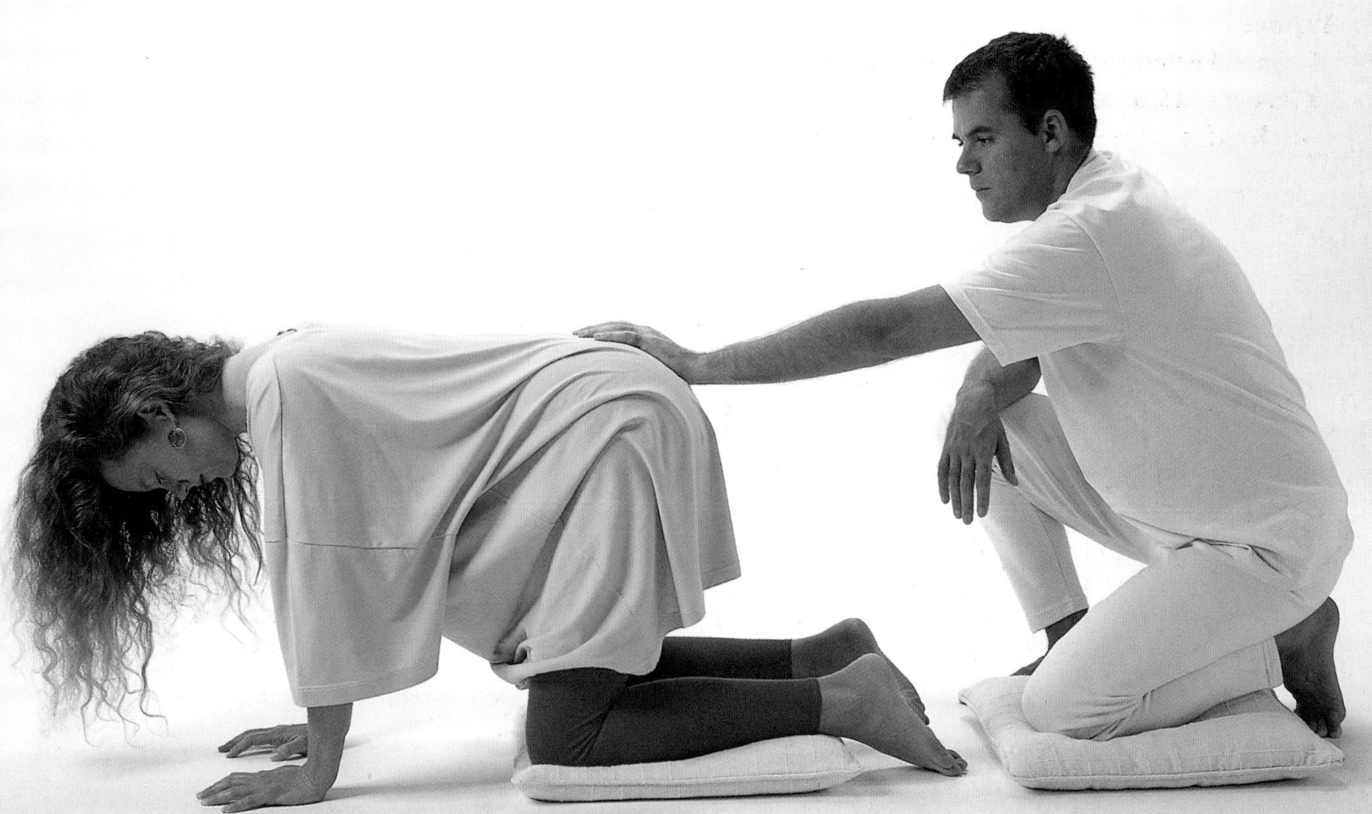

CIRCLING THE HIPS

1 Stand comfortably facing a wall. Fold your arms and place them on the wall, resting your head on your forearms, with your neck and shoulders relaxed.

2 As you inhale through your nose and exhale through your mouth, slowly rotate your hips. This is a position you may want to do in labor.

3 Let your partner know how the massage feels and if you'd like more pressure.

Partner

1 Stand comfortably beside your partner and rest the palm of one hand in the center of her lower back at the height of her waistline. Relax your arm and breathe evenly.

2 Tune in to her rhythm and then slowly massage down and around her lower back and hips, using a slow, continuous circular movement. Keep the pressure soft and even unless she asks you to massage more firmly.

3 Continue for a minute or so and then rest. Repeat once or twice.

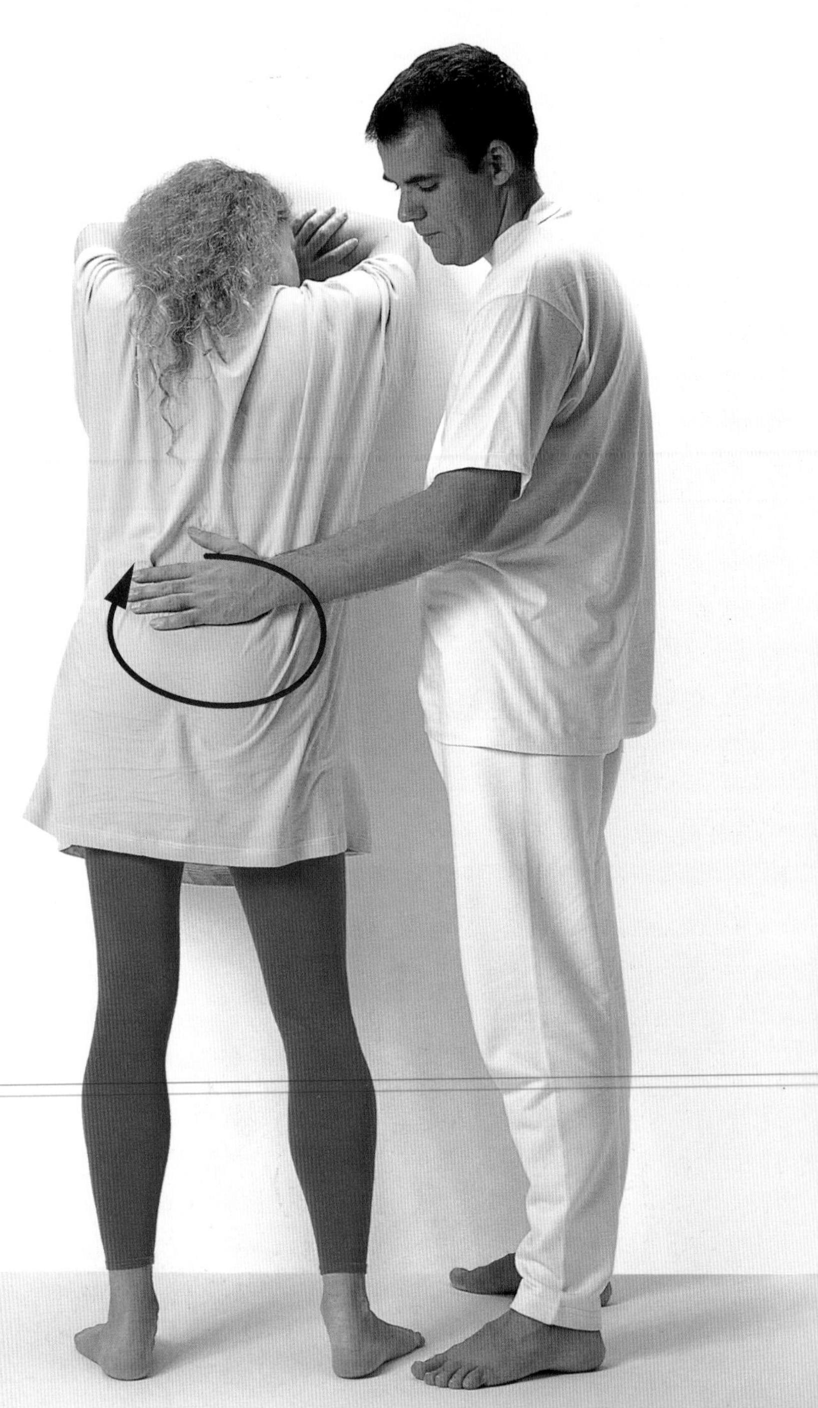

SIDE TO SIDE

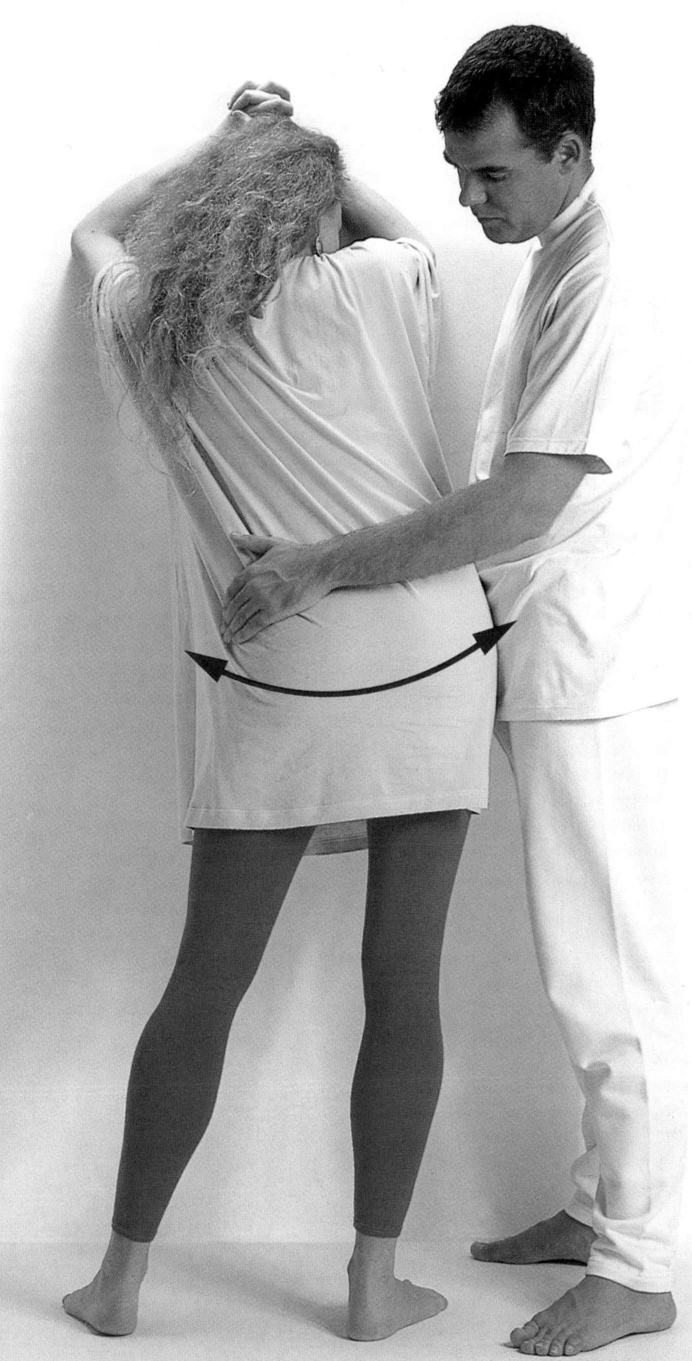

1 Stand comfortably facing a wall. Clasp your hands or fold your arms and place them on the wall, resting your head against them. Your neck and shoulders should be relaxed.

2 Swing your hips from side to side while breathing evenly.

3 Let your partner know how the massage feels.

Partner

1 Stand to the side of your partner, with your hand resting gently on her hip. Focus on your own breathing for a few seconds.

2 Tune in to her rhythm and then stroke across her lower back from side to side. Work in the opposite direction of her movements so that as she comes toward you, your hand moves away, and as she moves away, your hand comes toward you.

3 Continue doing this for a minute or so. Rest and repeat once or twice.

BABY AWARENESS

Focusing on the presence of your baby creates a feeling of peace and harmony—a perfect way to begin or end the exercise session. It is especially enjoyable to share the baby awareness exercise with your partner, giving him and your baby an opportunity to begin to get to know each other before the birth.

1 Make sure you are completely comfortable, lying in your partner's arms with your back supported. If you are working with another pregnant mother, sit back to back so that your lower back is in contact with hers and your spine feels free; fold your legs and put cushions under your knees. Close your eyes and let your hands rest softly on your partner's hands or on your belly.

2 Focus on your breathing, exhaling and inhaling in a comfortable rhythm. Let any feelings of tension or tightness in your body melt away. Feel your whole body becoming softer and more relaxed with each breath. Continue as in the BABY AWARENESS exercise on page 13.

Partner

1 If you are holding your partner, sit on a cushion with your back supported by a wall. Support your partner as she leans against you, making sure you are both comfortable.

2 Focus on the presence of your baby. Try to communicate with your baby by stroking your partner's belly with your hands or visualizing and talking inwardly to your baby.

3 Spend a minute or so resting and relaxing with your baby. Then very slowly bring your concentration back to your breathing, your body, and the room around you. Open your eyes and relax.

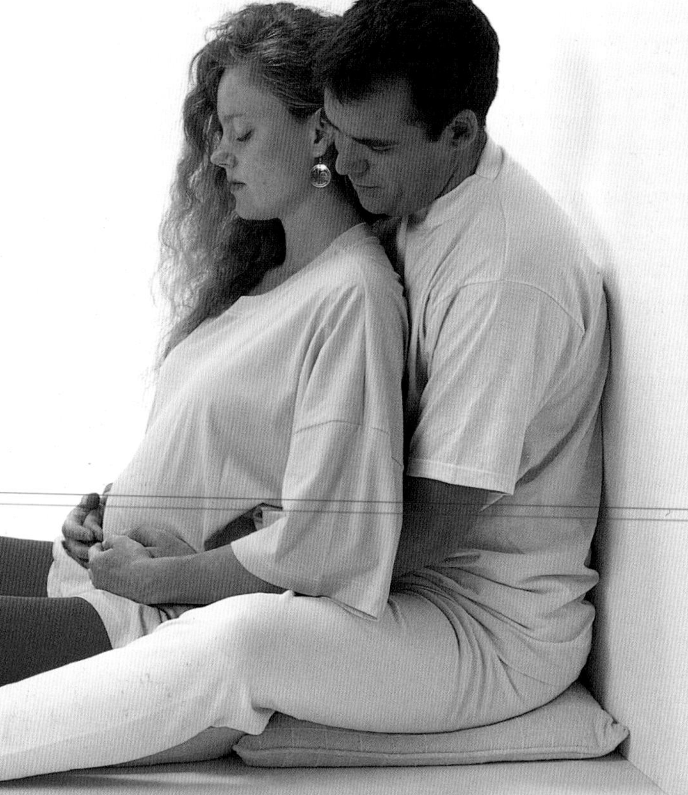

RELAXING MASSAGE

This is a wonderful way to end your session together. When done by two pregnant mothers working together, one begins massaging the other, and then they switch places. A couple can do this after a warm bath in the evening to help the pregnant mother have a peaceful sleep.

1 Lie on your right side first, with cushions under your head and supporting your left leg. You should be completely comfortable. Relax and breathe evenly, clearing your mind of all thoughts.

2 Let your body surrender to the support of the ground and the touch of your partner's hands, releasing and relaxing as you breathe.

3 Turn over when your partner has finished massaging your left side.

Partner

1 Kneel comfortably behind your partner, and place one hand on her hip and the other on the top of her shoulder. Massage her shoulder, her shoulder blade, and her neck, encouraging the muscles to relax and release.

2 Work down her upper and lower arm until you reach her hand. Then slowly massage her spine from top to bottom, pausing to work into any area that feels tight or tense.

3 Work down through her waistline to her lower back. Focus on the uppermost side of her lower back and on her top hip, and then continue down her top leg and foot unil you reach her toes.

4 Ask your partner to turn over onto her left side. Repeat the massage down the right side of her body.

5 Cover your partner with a warm blanket or towel to relax for a few minutes before you switch places.

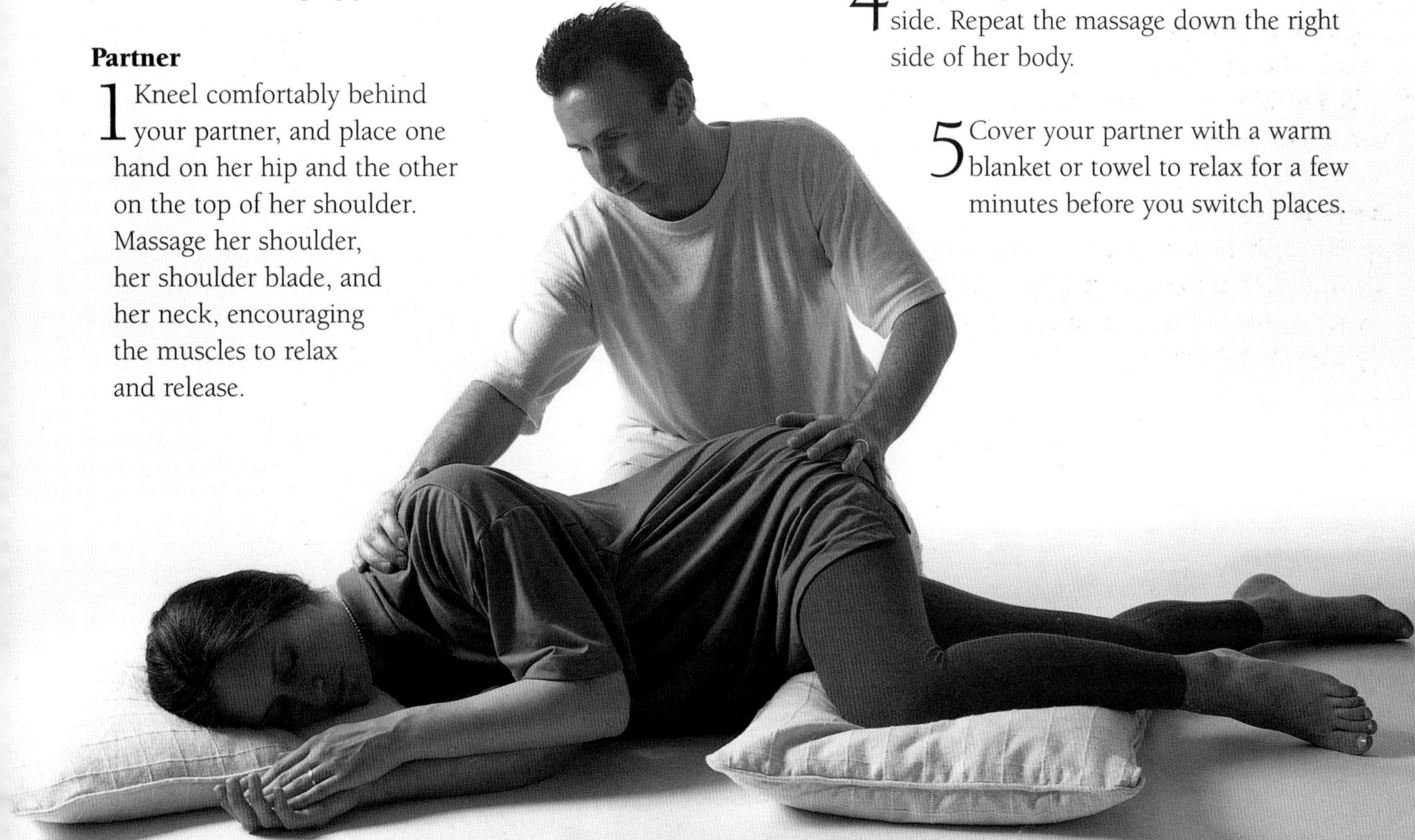

INDEX

FURTHER READING

Other useful works by Janet Balaskas that complement the pregnancy exercise system she has devised and reflect her approach to preparing for birth include: *New Active Birth* (Harvard Common Press), *The Encyclopedia of Pregnancy and Birth*, coauthor Yehudi Gordon (Little, Brown), and *Natural Pregnancy* (Interlink).

Author's Acknowledgments

I would like to thank Sylvia Bazzarelli, Marcus Dos Santos, Sarah Boyce, Naoko Chalkley, Jo Hamilton, Clare Harrison, Maureen Hibbert, Francesca Iliffe, Stephen Miller, Laila Mastenbrook, Julie Ann Miller, Harriet Mould, Juliette and Alan Stuart, Michelle Twiddy, Adrienne Wilkinson—the pregnant mothers and their partners from my classes who cheerfully posed for the lovely pictures that illustrate this book—and also Anthea Sieveking who photographed them so beautifully. Thanks also to my colleagues and fellow Active Birth Teachers who have participated in the evolution of the exercises, refining them with the benefit of our shared experience. I am also very grateful to Jean Sutton for her work on "Optimal Foetal Positioning," which has enabled me to revise and update the exercises so that pregnant mothers can use their bodies sensibly to encourage a problem-free and normal childbirth. Judy Hargreaves's wonderful work with couples and families. has inspired me to introduce into this program the communication exercises for partners to do together. This is my first book published by Frances Lincoln and I would like to thank everyone involved for making the creation of this book such an enjoyable experience.

Publishers' Acknowledgments

Editors Sarah Mitchell
Alison Freegard
Art editor Louise Kirby
Initial design Sally Cracknell
Designer Sara Robin
Editorial assistant Jon Folland
Production Jennifer Cohen
Index Hilary Bird

Editorial Director Erica Hunningher
Art Director Caroline Hillier

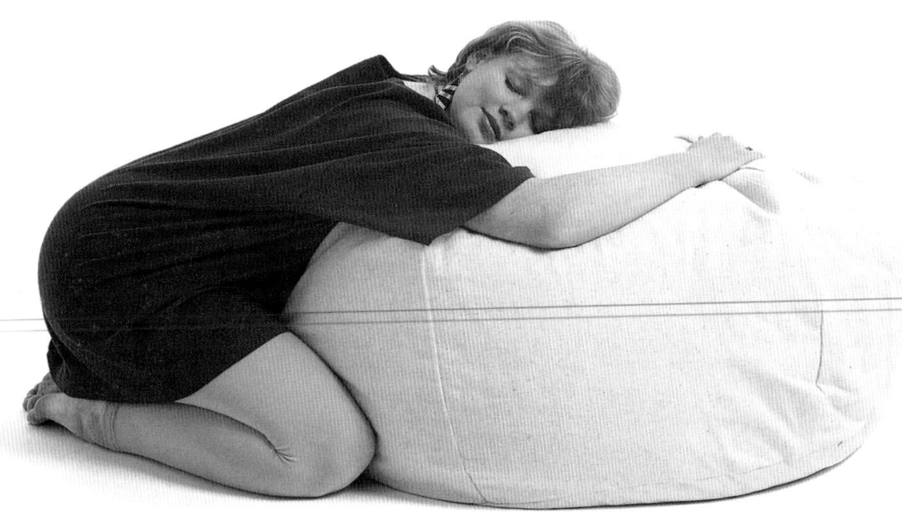